INCREASE YOUR HEIGHT and LOOSE YOUR WEIGHT

(A perfect guide for increasing height
and keeping your body slim and trim)

Published by :
Lotus Press Publishers & Distributors

INCREASE YOUR HEIGHT and LOOSE YOUR WEIGHT

(A perfect guide for increasing height and keeping your body slim and trim)

Dr. Rajeev Sharma

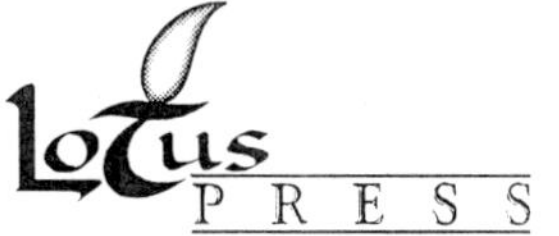

4735/22, Prakash Deep Building
Ansari Road, Darya Ganj,
New Delhi - 110002

Lotus Press : Publishers & Distributors
Unit No. 220, 2nd Floor, 4735/22, Prakash Deep Building,
Ansari Road, Darya Ganj, New Delhi- 110002
Ph.: 41355510, 98118-38000
• E-mail : lotuspress1984@gmail.com
www.lotuspress.co.in

Increase Your Height and Loose Your Weight

ISBN: 81-8382-164-2

Printed & Published by : **Lotus Press Publishers & Distributors**, New Delhi-02

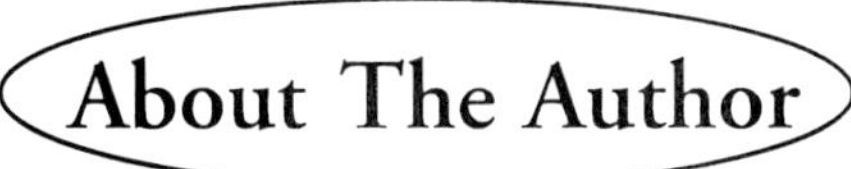

About The Author

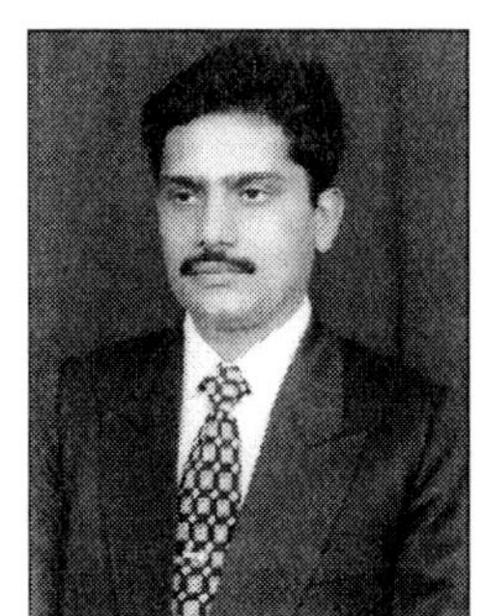

Dr. Rajeev Sharma

Dr. Rajeev Sharma is an eminent consultant of Homoeo-pathy, Yoga, Naturopathy and Alternative Medicine in India. He has written more than two hundred twenty five books (225) in Hindi and English and around one thousand articles which have been published in various newspapers and magazines. He is also an Editorial Board Member of the prestigious Asian Homoeopathic Journal besides many other newspapers and magazines.

Dr. Rajeev Sharma has written books on ayurveda, homoeopathy, yoga, naturopathy, accupressure, magnetotherapy, water-therapy, massage and aroma-therapy etc., and on all major ailments.

Dr. Rajeev Sharma is Medical Advisor to Ralson Remedies (a homoeopathic manufacturer), and Dixit Pharmacy (Ayurvedic Manufacturer), Sr. Medical Officer U.P. Govt. He has received several prizes for his outstanding achievements. He has been awarded the *Best Author Prize in Hindi* by the Ministry of Health and Family Welfare, Government of India and *Sarjana Puraskar* by *U.P. Hindi Sansthan*, Lucknow. He has delivered talks on All India Radio and Total T.V. and lectures on Alternative Medicine in various Government and Non-government Organisations. He has written Advt. Scripts for the products of several companies.

He has established an institute through which you can get certificates by correspondence in Accupressure, Massage, Yoga, Water Therapy, Diet Therapy, Naturopathy, Colour Therapy and Reiki besides other paramedical courses.

He is providing literature on Personality Development and Life-Style Management.

Dr. Rajeev Sharma is also a social activist. He has worked a lot against Addiction and Prevention of AIDS. He has worked for population and pollution control and human rights and has received the World Human Rights Promotion Award. His name has been published in *LIMCA BOOK OF RECORDS,* 2005. He has developed a website too :- www.newkamasutra.com

Dr. Rajeev Sharma is National President of an NGO UTKRISHTA BHARAT (An All India Association of Socio-Cultural-Religious and Sports Activities).

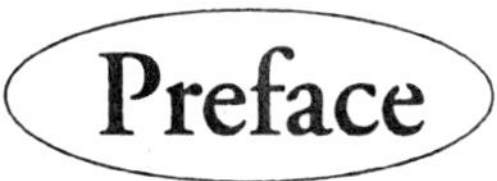

Every person wants to be tall and slim. But height depends on several factors and slimming depends on our life style.

As far as height is concerned no body can deny the fact that sufficient differences are visible in the castes, sub castes, tribes and families of the same country. Differences are also visible in the inhabitants of the different states within a country. It has been seen that tall and thin persons belonging to a single caste resemble their ancestors.

But from this inference you should not think that since your parents and ancestors are tall and strong, you will become tall automatically. If the growth of your stature is stopped, efforts should be made to reinforce the growth continuously. This book also helps in he same.

The child can grow properly during childhood under the supervision of its parents. The child, whose development takes place properly in the beginning, grows into a tall and well build adult. It can, therefore, be inferred that if the good, the attentive and the educated parents take proper care, their offspring can also grow into well build and tall adults.

For slimming, if you adopt the course, elaborated in this book, only for a few weeks to reduce ugly fat and weight, you can get success but you have to be careful about your weight for all the time. Often, people who undergo a slimming course complain that their weight went down in the beginning, but it again increased after some time and in the end they found themselves at the same point from where they started.

You must understand the reason for this. The main reason is that usually people are unable o change their habits. It is all the more true regarding dietary habits. You have to firmly resolve that you have to get rid of your obesity and excess weight, then only you can bring about remarkable changes in your habits. It is the will that matters. Excersises also play an important role.

In this book, I have tried to summarise all the diet plans and exercises along with yoga, helpful in increasing height and reducing weight.

I am very much thankful to Mrs. Neelima Kaushik in helping me in drawing of illustrations.

Hope, readers will be benefitted.

Dr. Rajeev Sharma

Srijan—Aarogya Jyoti®
Palm—11/03, Shipra Sun City
Ghaziabad (U.P.)
Ph.: 0120-6460127
email: sharmarajeev108@rediffmail.com

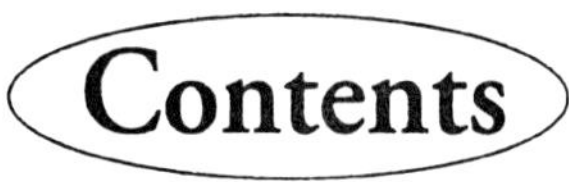
Contents

HEIGHT

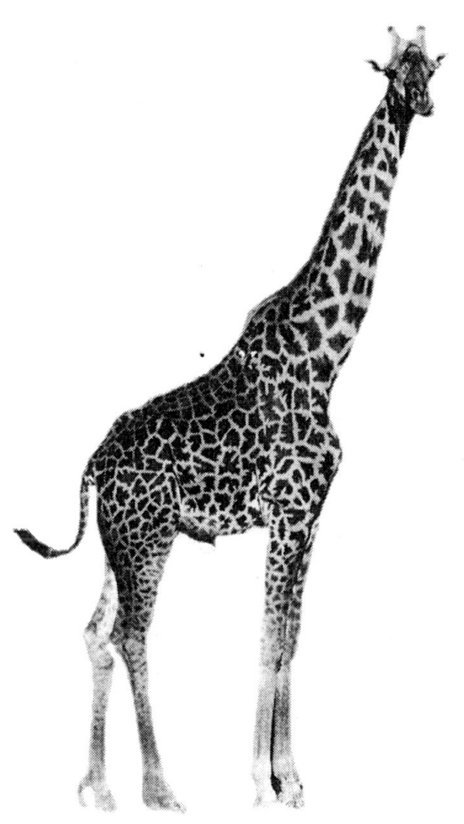

1

Short Stature—A Curse

Many years ago (in the seventh decade of the 20th century) the dwarfs started a country-wide movement in Australia to provide good facilities for themselves. The short-statured people of Australia and New Zealand had participated in it by coming from every nook and corner. Their parents, too, participated in this conference to tell the people about the hardships and difficulties which their sons and daughters had to face on account of their short statures. The chairman of the conference, Whitker, who himself was a short-statured person (dwarf), told the participants that on account of being short-statured, they had to experience many difficulties in getting employment. The result was that they had become a redundant part of society.

The curse of short stature is being experienced very seriously in every corner of the world. Be it business, or high government service, only tall persons or candidates of average height are selected for the jobs. Tall stature has almost become an important condition for selection in I.P.S., Air Force, Navy or in some other jobs. On several occasions, even in a personal sphere, short-stature stands in the way of getting a suitable partner in life of one's own choice. Several examples have come to light in France, Britain and America, where the beloved refused to marry a youngman who had a short stature. Such cases are also there when a beautiful woman had to wait for the whole of her life for marriage due to short stature.

What is the Ideal Height?

There has been a difference of opinion in different countries and at different times, regarding the ideal heights of men and women. The height is very much related to the climate of a country and also to the heredity of a person.This is the reason why the standards differ from one country to another.There is one standard in Greece, another in Europe and quite different from these in America. So the standard varies in Asia. The standard in India is different from that of Iran, while the standards of China and Japan are quite different from these.

In England, France and America, the average height of a man varies from five feet to six feet and four inches, while the average height of ladies varies from four feet nine inches to six feet. In Asia, the average height of an Indian is slightly below the average height of European countries, while the height in China and Japan is much less than what you find in India.

The artists, the artisans and the scientists also differ very much from each other regarding the conception of 'Ideal Height'. The scientists lay great emphasis upon the development of physique, but the artists lay greater emphasis on 'beauty' and 'symmetry'. In our opinion, both the views are correct and have their own importance. Hence both the points of view have to be kept in sight while planning to increase one's height.

The Greek standard is that the height of a man should be eight times the length of his head. The modem artists point out that the stature of a man should be seven and a half times the length of his head.

If the length of the head of a man is nine inches, his height should be five feet and ten and a half inches. This is called the ideal height of a man according to the Greek standard. In the same proportion, the height of a woman is considered to be ideal if it is five feet and five and a half inches. The form or shape of the arms, hands, and, thighs and feet should also be in the same proportion.

■

2

Inhibiting Factors to Height-Gain

There are multiple and variable factors that prove as impedimental causes in inhibiting height, as listed below:

(a) Psychological
(b) Dietary aspect
(c) Society and family impact
(d) Physical disabilities, diseases
(e) Financial Problems
(f) Lack of Physical activity
(g) Burden of studies
(h) Pollution and Environmental hazards
(i) Heredity and genetic factor

In all persons whose growth is retarded, it is not necessary that all the forementioned factors could be found/traced commonly but in majority of cases of this type, there could definitely be one or more of such causes. Which have impacted a child or adolescent's growth prospects.

Psychological Factors

In most of the Indian homes, especially in the rural and traditional homes, girl is still considered to be a burden. She is neither provided with nutritional diet, nor with proper education, rather she is employed as a tool to serve rest of the members in the family. Her personal needs and care are thrown to winds and is humiliated even by males younger to her. Such a neglected girl cannot ventilate her grievances, demand even bare minimum things, ask for little favours, complain against her brothers or any other dominant male/female member. She is expected to cater to needs of all the family members but is denied the right to demand anything. Not only male but even females also give her a cold shoulder. At the age of puberty, the adolescent girl has to herself encounter all the menstrual, physical and psychological problems. In her quest for a viable solution she has to run for advice to outsiders or else is misled.

All the said factors cripple her mental and physical progress, her body doesn't grow at a pace at which it should normally grow. She feels neglected and such a condition is exploited, economically or sexually, by others. If her mother, is a stepmother it will further add to her woes. Such a girl prefers to stay away from home on one pretext or the other. All such unfavourable episodes impact her whole life pattern. If you ever come across such a girl, you can easily notice anguish, frustration and feeling of negligence upon her face and expressions. Even a sympathy drives her to wrong hands and she is exploited.

The parents are reminded that if they treat their daughters as second grade creatures and discriminate against them, fail to fulfil even their genuine demands, scuttle their hopes and aspirations, deny them the right and opportunity to study, hurt abuses on them, deride and demean them, they are simply committing a heinous social crime, if not a Sin.

All know that today's girl is tomorrow's wife and mother but, if her childhood is disturbed with the aforesaid discrimination, her mental and physical growth is bound to get retarded—much to the detriment of the girl, her family members and (rather) society as a whole. If you want a happy family, accord respect to the female child, look to her multiple problems, try to address yourself to her problems and try to meet her, at least, genuine and tenable demands. Do not strangulate her hopes and aspirations, rather help her in her all round progress and development. Remember, a happy, well educated, properly guided, nutritive fed, mentally bolstered up girl is a boon to society at large.

If parents assume the status of a police person, they will be committing the same blunder if they are too lenient and relenting. They have resort to a middle path, as too much pampering and too much of iron discipline are two ends of the same thread. A child's mental and physical growth will also get retarded if the children are treated with tough approach.

Psychological upsets and barriers can be easily by passed if parents give sufficient time to their siblings to express their views, ventilate their grievances, resolve their problems, satiate their inquisitiveness, meet their just and tenable demands, help them in their studies, have reasonable tab over their movements and the company they keep (but they ought not to be spied), how they spend pocket money. If the parents can educate, motivate, guide, persuade their children to see reason and appreciate their (parents) problems, they will be able to keep their children away from many ills— it will also keep their minds free from unnecessary burden, thus affording them greater opportunity to put in better performance. It will also ensure their multifaceted growth. To possess a balanced personality, mental alertness and presentable physique and normal height are the prerequisites of an all-round best personality. Handsome is that handsome does. Nobody will notice your presence or feel impressed by your physical figure, unless you are mentally alert and physically fit. To be a successful person one must be brilliant in all walks of life.

Dietary aspect and Growth

If your mind as at rest and free from worries and anxieties, you will relish even the most cost-effective and simple food and all digestive enzymes will intermingle with the masticated food to give essential energy to the body, by generating requisite energy. In a mentally agitated state even the costliest food will spoil your digestion.

Diet is the most difficult and intricate aspect which needs to be studied in greater details. A balanced diet is not necessarily the best suited diet nor the best diet is a balanced diet, as each body chemistry of each person is different and reacts differently in various situations.

Experts have worked out weight in relation to age and built of body but the tables are, by no means, the final word in this regard, as there are many other factors which are held responsible for proper or improper growth. A suitable balance sheet can be drawn to arrive at a decision, whether a person meets the set-forth standards. In ·any case, close relation between height and weight and weight and diet cannot be denied. Readers may study the given tables on age, weight and height and decide, for themselves, if they suitably measure up to the worked out standards.

Calories

Before we enter into various aspects of balanced diet, it is necessary to know what is implied by the word 'CALORIE'. Whatever food item generated certain amount of energy which is necessary for normal functions of various body parts (rather the body as a whole) when food generates energy, it must be expended (spent up) failing which it will result in various disorders. Hence, there is a close relationship between energy (Calorie) generation and spending. If requisite energy is not generated by intake of food and the body is taxed and overworked beyond its sustainable capacity, it will render the body weak and exhausted, resulting in a run-down condition. Conversely, if too much energy is generated but not expended, it will also result in disorders like obesity, diabetes, heart and respiratory problems, deprived digestion, immobility of body organs etc.

Calories are closely related to physical activity. For instance, a person doing hard and strenuous labour will require high calorie diet to meet the demands of his body. A growing child, pregnant and lactating mother; an elderly person, a sedentary person, a bed-ridden patient will, naturally require different calories. In order to maintain a suitable balance between energy generation and subsequent expension, diet must conform to the ratio between energy generation and expension. This is the only reason as to why different calorie-based diets have been worked out and suggested on the basis of nature of one's job, in relation to physical activity, for which tables given on subsequent pages may be studied.

Society and Family Impact

Everyone has to follow certain norms and disciplines practised and followed in a particular society, as man is a social animal and, thus, cannot easily revolt against such limitations and sanctions imposed. Changes are brought about through a revolt or resistance, as no society will permit its members to defy or disobey its rules.

When elderly discipline is imposed on growing children they wish to revolt but cannot ventilate their disagreement and, thus, it proves as an inhibitory factor in their growth spurt. The position is further compounded when elders force their children to abide by family discipline, without providing them an opportunity to ventilate their dissent. All such events lead to a sense of dissatisfaction and mental brooding. The children exhaust their energy in suppressing their desires.

In certain families disputes between parents, parents and grandparents, grown up and young children, inter-family disputes hurt a child immensely, resulting in his retarded growth and disturbed studies. Not only his mental fibre is shattered but his physical development also gets impacted. The parents and other elderly persons must ensure a hassle free and congenial atmosphere in the family for all round health of all family members.

Tips for Parents

- They should resist from discussing any dispute in the presence of their children.
- Should not expect their children to be partners in day-to-day problems.

- Should encourage their children to settle their problems by themselves.
- Induce and motivate them to abide by and follow at least laudable and time-tested norms and discipline.
- To live within social norms and respect feelings of others.
- To give them reasonable opportunity for growth of body, mind and intellect.
- To devote enough attention to their individual problems and give them a patient listening and try to amicably solve their problems.
- Do not burden their children with their personal, financial and social problems.

The young ones should feel free to approach their parents and other experienced persons to ventilate their grievances but they must not be derided, reprimanded or thrashed, snubbed or demeaned in the presence of other members. Personal interaction is the core factor in family happiness and general well-being.

Physical Disability and Diseases

Any disability like mental retardation, slow comprehension, blindness, curvature of bones, atrophied kidneys, wrinkled skin and senile look, clubbed foot, pigeon chest, curved and distorted face, rough and choked voice, hunched back, stooped shoulders, spastic·gait are some of the abnormalities which impact a person psychologically and, thus, mentally wreck him, as a result of which one is bound to suffer from inferiority complex and other such upsets. No doubt, all these are termed under 'disabilities' but are also liable to adversely affect his growth pattern. When a growing child is not accepted in the society, he becomes a social recluse and prefers to stay indoors, thus sacrificing his physical activity.

Apart from the said lengthy list of disabilities, fuel will be added to fire if he suffers also from short stature, tuberculosis, asthma, any skin disorder, some sort of urinary problem, soft tissue related disorders, bone deformities and/or curvature, flat nose, small neck. A growing girl hesitated to attend to her classes because she was suffering from acne and dark complexion while the other one shirked company as she was both obese and short statured, even though financially better off than her counterparts.

All the unsavoury, uncharitable invectives damage the affected person enormously and personality as a whole is shattered. It is the duty of the parents to give co-operation, support, and reassure to the child and help him/her in overcoming psychological barriers. Most of such abnormalities can be easily won over and managed by devoting more time to studies, indoor physical activity (like yoga, pranayama, aerobics, work up exercises). The teachers, coaches, well-wishers should endeavour to build up self-confidence and will power of such children and once you succeed, there won't be any going back. No doubt, some of the deformities cannot be managed even by best efforts and intentions, but what is manageable must be managed in a sensible way. If a child has any type of physical deformity, never call him by that name (For instance Lame, blind, blind of one eye etc). If parents and other housemates start calling by such names, outsiders will be free to tease that child.

Financial Problems

This aspect is closely related to income and if the earning member is only one, the problem is bound to get confused. A child, whose parents have limited income, can neither be served with growth related diet, nor given education in a prestigious school, nor even his minimum and reasonable demands met. When all these factors combine together, his alround growth will get impeded. His growth-related endocrine glands will continue to malfunction, resulting in inferiority complex, frail and weak body structure, short height, low IQ, diet deficient in essential nutrients. Such a deprived child will shun company, remain closed within the house, not take part in any sports related games, will be hesistant in approaching his teachers and classmates. Nothing much can be possibly done when financial crunch is the cause but the child's self-confidence can be restored and built up in a sustained manner. Here, the parents and teachers have to adopt a conciliatory, sympathetic and reassuring approach so that the child doesn't suffer from inferiority complex. Such children may be intellectuals but their physical growth is retarded. All persons are not financially sound; hence the child should mix up with his equals only, and stay away from the company of elite class children. He should mix up freely and participate in games and sports, ingest cheaper food items which are equally rich in nutrients (For instance carrots can be substituted for costly apples, cane sugar juice for costly products etc.)

Mental happiness is to be found more in less privileged children, as they gradually learn to channelise their energies in more constructive ways. Time is the best teacher and nature helps everyone to stay happy even in adverse financial situations.

Lack of Physical Activity

This is a syndrome of elite class children who do not play any outdoor sports nor for any activity where body is required to be exerted. Such children remain indoors, play only indoor games which are best of any vigorous activity, remain glued to T.V. and Video games, playing cards, carrom etc. They mix up with and enjoy company of those children who follow their habits.

These children are pampered ones, served by servants, do not perform even their normal work themselves, eat a lot either in their homes or outside, but perform no or very little activity to keep their bodies in good shape. They generally complain of one ailment or the other, have constipated bowels, suffer from bulk of digestion related problems, get exhausted even on minimum effort. Neither they themselves take to any physical activity nor are prevailed upon by their elders. Provision and abundant use of modern means of comfort suffice to turn them sloth, indolent and lazy. As a rule, a child must not avoid physical exertion except when there is some physical or mental inhibitory factor. Gradually such children turn obese and often fall a prey to digestive, respiratory, cardiac and locomotor disorders.

Such children are advised to do as suggested below or they should be pursuaded by their elders who should first themselves set an example and then advise or induce their kids.

- Get up early in the morning and go out for a brisk walk.
- Attend to their daily chores themselves but not to depend upon others to do the jobs for them.
- Should earmark morning or evening time for outdoor games.
- Eat only when really hungry, but must abstain from eating every now-and-then.
- Avoid remaining glued to T.V., video games and video movies.
- Take meals at home only but avoid taking anything outside home.
- Should perform Pranayama, preferably in the morning and also jumping, skipping, yogic, long and deep breathing exercises.
- Avoid using car, scooter/mobike or a cycle, even to cover a short distance. They must cultivate the habit of walking on foot.
- Involve themselves in domestic activities and help their housemates.
- Shouldn't sleep during day, or study or do any sort of serious studies after taking lunch. They may have a short nap or simply relax in an easy-chair.
- Shouldn't sleep immediately after taking meals, rather go out for a stroll. Remember, morning walk should be brisk and evening walk only a stroll.

- Avoid watching T.V or listening to Radio while taking meals. Devote full attention to your meals and try to relish your food.
- In case of any illness, resort to only moderate physical activity but never over strain your system.

It is repeated that whatever we eat should not normally cause any sort of upset. When we go on overloading our digestive system with food, our body cannot derive any benefit. The best way to keep fit and healthy is a sensible balance between diet and exercise, and dietary intake must conform to the quantum of energy expended. If you generate higher calories but do no or negligible physical activity, one is able to hinder his growth. If there is more of physical activity but is not suitably compensated by requisite food intake, it will also spoil health. So, eat only that much is actually required by your body neither less or more than what is actually needed.

Even if a child is having an ideal height but his body is obese, he will look short statured; conversely if a person is tall and slim but his body is lean, he will look odd. Height must commensurate with weight and such a situation can only be maintained if there is a proper balance between diet and exercise. If you opt to sacrifice one aspect for the other, you are simply inviting a Calamity/problem.

Burden of Studies

Burden of studies is so much on the young kids that rest, exercise and diet are relegated to the hind seat. The parents not only unduly tax their kids but also commit the blunder of comparing them with other children, especially those of relatives and friends. Mad race for higher marks doesn't let the parents and their children enjoy rest. Burden of hometask so heavily weighs on a child that he can neither eat nor take rest. Immediately after serving meals, the innocent children are burdened and coaxed to devote more time to studies. 'Public School Syndrome' and 'Comparing one's own children with other children' makes the parents blind to requirements and necessities of childhood. Children lose peace of mind, sacrifice rest and comfort, forego even meals, overburden their minds and bodies simply to satiate their parents mad hankering for high score results.

If a child goes on studying doesn't eat well, but is denied even reasonable rest, not allowed to play any game, is confined within four walls and not allowed to interact with his class-mates, his all-round development is bound to get adversely affected. Neither he will develop physically nor mentally, rather he will become a prisoner in his own home.

The parents must mend their ways and thinking process. By studying more and putting in extra hours in study, children do not become eligible for securing more marks and put in better performance. It is a wrong and misplaced notion and injudicious approach to overburden a child with studies. This is a fad and obsession which the parents must give up at the earliest opportunity. The parents will not gain if their children fall ill, become recluse, divorce their physical activity and also are unable to eat well. Remember good and nutritious diet, proper and regular physical activity, mental peace, physical and mental relaxation, requisite rest and sleep are the prerequisites for any child's all-round development and progress. Weak eye-sight, backache, pain in neck and shoulders, agitated behaviour are some of the fall-out symptoms of overstudy.

Give reasonable freedom to your child as far as mode and timing of study is concerned, but never force him against his will, rather give him the freedom to adjust his, timings as he chooses. But that doesn't mean that he should waste time or skip his study and playtime.

Engaging teachers at home or in Coaching Centres is not a matter of necessity but a sheer pseudo status symbol. If your child attends to his classes regularly and does his homework daily, there is hardly any need for extra study and coaching. In any case, never burden you child by persistently getting on his nerves to over strain himself, thereby spoiling his health and disturbing peace of mind.

Pollution and Environmental Hazards

Pollution does not directly impact a child's growth but, all the same, is decidedly a potent factor in damaging his health. Air, noise and water pollutions are quite common in big towns and metros. Allergy, asthma, skin, nose, throat, mouth are the general types of pollutions. Polluted water is a common source of many gastrointestinal disorders. Sneezing, cough, asthma, bronchitis, hypersensitivity of skin, loose motions/constipation are some of the known symptoms. Noise pollution is held responsible for hard of hearing, deafness and other auditory disorders. Not only children but almost all the elders are also equally affected by pollution.

The children should be encouraged to go to green fields, gardens, lakes, rivers, ponds and open areas where air is not polluted. Even a 5-minute daily course of deep-breathing will suffice to generate renewed energy, let in oxygen and let out poisonous gases. Fresh air and fresh water are indispensible for a healthy living. I am not elaborating on this aspect more, since people are fully conscious of environmental hazards.

Heredity and Genetic Factor

Height in certain races is genetically short. For instance, in Yellow/Manchurian races where both boys and girls are short-statured, because their parents are also short, though this genetic factor, at times, belies the truth, and exceptions, though quite glaring, are still not non-existent. Similarly, in Europe and America parents are quite tall and some of whom are even abnormally tall and, in 8 out of 10 cases, their siblings are also tall in accordance with their age.

■

3

The Foundation of One's Stature is Laid in Childhood

The child can grow properly during its childhood under the supervision of its parents. The child whose development takes place properly in the begining, grows into a tall and well build adult. It can, therefore, be inferred that if the good, the attentive and the educated parents take proper care, their offspring can also grow into well build and tall adults.

Undoubtedly, all the parents want that their children may become tall and possess an attractive personality. But only those parents can achieve their goal, who can back their desires with the right type of efforts.

You may ask a hundred times as to what is this effort, but our reply will be one and the same. While the child is in the growing stage, take every possible care to bring it up properly. Put your child in the open on a mat and afford it an opportunity to move its hands and legs freely, while lying on its back.

If the ground on which the child is lying down is hard and even, it will be able to do bodily exercise by moving its hands and legs. Thus while it grows into an adult, its body will become proportionate, soft and modifiable.

Student Period and the Evil Effects of Wrong Posture

In countries like India, when the children grow, they usually go to school. The children of average parents (who get admission in Government Schools) usually come again in an unwholesome atmosphere. They are kept together in a school. In the classrooms there is usually an insufficient light and in many cases no desks are provided to the children to work. And even in the institutions where desks are provided, they are often smaller than the size of children. Besides, there is insufficient light and air. Such an unnatural atmosphere casts an unwholesome effect on the development of a child. The bones are flexible during childhood., This is the age when the body grows. In such a condition, the necks of children often bend on one side and there appears to be a hunch in their backs and their waists also shrink inwards. The knees of several children start bending downwards and the sides of the backbone develop unnatural curves.

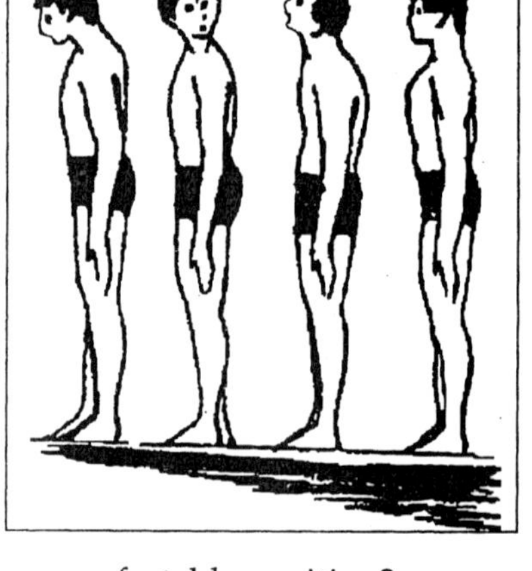

When the wrong posture becomes a part of the nature of a child, the development of his body, when, he comes of age, does not take place properly. Those amongst you, who have become short-statured on account of bad posture should ascertain the following:

1. Did you not sleep in your childhood with your brothers and sisters on a single bed in an uncomfortable position?
2. Did you not sleep on a small bed so that you had cultivated the habit of bending your legs while sleeping?
3. Have you not developed the habit of sitting in a crouch position?
4. Did you not develop the habit of leaning forward while walking, in your student days, due to heavy load of your school bag?
5. Did you not lean forward while reading?
6. Did you not take adequate part in games in your school?
7. Have you not cultivated the habit of reading while lying in bed?

You will find that most of these defects existed in you. We would like to add here that if you are short-statured or your posture is defective, or your personality is not attractive, there is one reason for all these shortcomings, that you have cultivated wrong habits, on account of which your stature has remained short, or if it is not short, it looks short.

The only remedy to improve your height is that you should bring improvement within yourself even at this stage and try to give up the bad old habits, gradually.

Smoking and your Stature

In the opinion of a physiologist of Chicago, tobacco contains nicotine, which is so poisonous that if 1/400 oz. of it is injected into the blood of a man, he will die. One third part of this quantity is always present in each cigarette. The heartbeat increases due to nicotine. The heart of a smoker has to beat 30,000 times in twenty-four hours. From this, it is gathered that nicotine is a poisonous substance. Due to constant smoking slow poison accumulates in the body. The lungs are consequently affected and digestion is also disturbed. The rickets of the chest increase and memory is also affected.

The cigarettes contain certain poisonous elements, which very much hinder the development of the body, particularly during adolescence. Smoking not only badly affects the lungs of a person, but there is always a fear of 'cancer' and the growth of the stature is also retarded. This is the conclusion which is derived from the latest scientific researches. Al the scientists also agree with the inference that the nicotine present in cigarettes is very much harmful for health. Hence the people who want to increase their height are advised to get rid of this habit as early as possible.

■

4

How does the Length of the Various Parts of the Body Increase or Decrease?

The structure of any part of our body is closely related to its function. If the function of any organ changes, then its structure will also undergo a change. Conversely, if the structure of any part undergoes a change, its function also changes. If a man takes exercise every day, the muscles of those parts of the body, which perform the relevant movements, become strong. The more you take work from an organ, the form and shape of the muscles of that organ gets enlarged proportionately and they also become strong. On the contrary, the muscles of those organs of the body which are not used, are gradually reduced in size and even their natural form slowly disappear.

Our Body and its Structure

The structure of the human body is very complex. Our body is made of innumerable cells. These cells are divided into a number of groups which are called tissues. Certain tissues form the external surface of the body while others join other tissues. Some tissues go to form 'muscles' while others form 'nerves'. An organ is formed by a group of tissues. These organs can be made strong and be developed by giving proper exercise and movements to them.

As you are aware, there are nine main organ systems in our body. Their brief descriptions are given below:

(1) *The Skeletal System*—It provides the skeleton for the body. There are many bones in it, whose joints are interconnected with several connecting tissues. Thus a man can direct the various movements of his body. The back-

bone has a special place in the human skeleton. (It is also closely related to the stature of a man.)

(2) *The Muscular System*—Its function is to help in the performance of movements of the different parts of the human body such as head, neck, arms, trunk, legs etc. It performs the function of blood circulation and sends the food in the food pipe of the body. All the activities of our body are governed by this system.

(3) *The Digestive System*—Its function is to digest the food which generates energy. (The undigested food is also passed out in the form of stool through this system.)

(4) *The Respiratory System*—To get energy from the food that is digested, oxygen is necessary. This system helps in the procurement of oxygen. It also helps our body to send out carbon dioxide gas from it.

(5) *The Circulatory System*—This system is responsible for sending the energy procured from the nourishing elements of our food and the oxygen procured from the air, to all the parts of the body. All the cells of our body require energy and oxygen. Its circulation takes place through blood. The blood, the blood vessels and the heart—all three combine to form this system.

(6) *The Excretory System*—Its main function is to send out the refuse and the useless matter out of our body. The kidneys, ureter and urinary bladder form this system. (The urine is passed out through this system.) Other parts of the body also assist in sending out the waste matter e.g. perspiration from the skin and sending out carbon dioxide gas from the lungs.

(7) *The Reproductive System*—The organs which form this system are different in men and women. The reproductive organ of the male consists of the penis and the testes, while reproductive organ of the female consists of ovaries, uterus and other parts.

(8) *The Nervous System*—It exercises a check over the functions of the different parts of human body. The brain, spinal chord and the nerves form this system.

(9) *The Endocrine System*—'Endocrine' means secreting internally. This system mainly consists of certain glands, which secrete fluids, which get directly mixed up in the blood. These secretions are called 'hormones' and the glands secreting them are also called 'ductless glands'. The important glands are thyroid, adrenal, pituitary and the pancreas. Though there are several systems in our body, yet all of them function together. The thyroid gland is mainly connected with the development of the body and the stature of a person. We will discuss it in brief in' the next step.

The Thyroid Gland and Your Stature

Yes, as we have already told you the thyroid gland is an endocrine gland on account of which the hormone directly mixes with the blood. It is a ductless gland.

The thyroid gland is associated with the weight of a person. On the basis of recent researches, the experts have arrived at the conclusion that the activity of the thyroid gland creates an unprecedented increase in the height of a person in young age. Nevertheless, it is true that in the phenomenon of increase in stature, other glands too have their role to play. Even then this can be definitely stated that if this gland does not function properly, the development is not normally possible.

According to experts, "It is very difficult to study the general functions of this gland in an average individual. To understand its function, the best course is to observe the defects which are found (in a human organism) when this gland does not function properly or when it is removed from the body of a person. In that condition, the growth of the bones is stopped or the bones are deformed or mis-shaped. The sexual maturity of a person becomes slow or is stopped. The skin becomes dry. The muscles grow weak and fatigue occurs. Not only this, the development of the body stops, the stature remains short and a growing body too tends to become short."

From the study of the above defects, one thing becomes very clear that the thyroid gland affects all the cells of the body and, therefore, it is very significant.

Now let us look at its reverse. If the thyroid gland becomes hyperactive, the result will be just different. The heart-beat increases, the appetite increases all at once, but after having taken food in an unusual quantity, the person becomes dull all of a sudden. The person feels great energy and enthusiasm in him, and becomes very much restless. The skin becomes moist. The temperature of the body increases, and the quantity of glucose in it becomes more than normal.

It need not be said, that the claim of increasing the height can be made in such circumstances, but the person should be treated by an expert physician, otherwise the desired results will not be forthcoming.

In the nineteenth century, there were many fields in the inland regions, which were called 'Goitre Zones', for the inhabitants of such places mostly suffered from the hypo-activity of the thyroid glands. They were administered iodine, which led to the disappearance of the disease, and their normal growth began again in its natural form.

If you are anxious to increase your height, follow our course according to the technique outlined and you will find that you have improved a lot and you are on the path of progress.

The Backbone

In the backbone of the human body, there are 33 vertebrae. Each vertebra has a hole in it, resembling a ring. The vertebrae are joined together and form a continuous hollow tube in which the spinal chord is lodged. The vertebral column can be divided into five parts: (1) The Cervical Region (2) The

Thoracic Region (3) The Lumbar Region (4) The Sacral Region and (5) The Coccyx Region.

The upper-most part of the vertebral column forms the part of the neck which has seven vertebrae. The first and the second vertebra of the neck are joined in such a way that we can move our head in any direction that we like—forward or backward, towards the right or the left. The second part of the vertebral column is called the Thoracic Region. There are 12 vertebrae in it. The third part is called the Lumbar Region. The vertebrae present in this part are long and heavy. There are 5 vertebrae in it. The fourth part is called the Sacral Region. There are 5 vertebrae in it, which are separate from each other at the time of birth. Later they get joined together and take the shape of a bone in a triangular form known as Sacrum. The fifth part is called the Coccyx Region. It has 4 vertebrae, which after sometime join with each other and form a Coccyx.

The backbone has a very important position in our body. It is not only the backbone of the body, but it is also the backbone of the health of a man. The stature of the man is very much related to the vertebral column. If the backbone functions properly, the man enjoys good health. Usually when people feel pain in the back, or in the waist, they become anxious.

If we do not perform movements prescribed for the backbone regularly and become careless in looking after our body, and also adopt a defective posture while sitting, the backbone will develop certain curvatures. When these curvatures increase, the stature will become short and several other defects will follow. These defects can be easily removed only by a regular practice of the movements prescribed.

There is a spongy cushion like structure in between two vertebrae, which protects them from getting rubbed against each other, while they are in motion. When this cushion comes out from its proper place or is dislocated, there is pain in them. In that condition, one has to go to the orthopaedic surgeon and get the dislocated cushion set in its proper place.

In order to ensure that the vertebrae and the cushions function properly, the backbone should be massaged daily with oil. This will not only make the vertebral column healthy, but also lead to its development.

Selection of Clothes

People of average stature and physique should neither put on very tight clothes nor those very loose. But fat people can be advised to put on a little tight clothes so that their corpulence may be slightly checked. From this it follows that the directions too can vary according to changing circumstances. If fat people put on loose dresses, their corpulence can further increase.

There are certain people whose legs are smaller as compared to the upper portion of their bodies. Conversely, there are people whose legs are longer and the upper portion of their bodies is smaller. In case you want to show the upper portion of your body longer than the lower, you can put on an open shirt or have your shirt outside your pant. Similarly, those people whose legs are smaller, but who want to show their lower portion taller can do so by putting their shirts inside their pants.

On contrary, there are some ladies who are unusually tall. If they do not want to show themselves very tall, they should put on loose dresses. This would make their stature look a bit shorter.

■

5

Improve Your Posture Improve Your Height

Meaning of the word posture is to find out the position in which you keep the different parts of your body while rising, sitting, walking, running or lying down. Keeping the various parts of your body in a proper position or maintaining a correct posture is as much essential for the development of your body, as it is for making your gait look beautiful and your personality attractive.

The development of the different parts of one's body takes place in the mother's womb. Sometimes, the child grows in the womb in a defective position and the structure of the various parts of the body becomes faulty. These physical deformities can be set right with the help of a doctor.

When a man or a woman crosses the adolescent period, his or her appearance and posture assume a specific pattern. His or her personality starts developing. Right posture makes a person impressive, which enables him or her to create a name for himself or herself. On the other hand, the personality of man whose posture is defective becomes gloomy and dull. Wherever he goes, he avoids company and starts losing confidence in himself. Thus your posture creates a definite effect on your personality.

You can Improve Your Posture

Quite a number of persons amongst you may ask if they could rectify the wrong positions of their body; or if they could correct their posture.

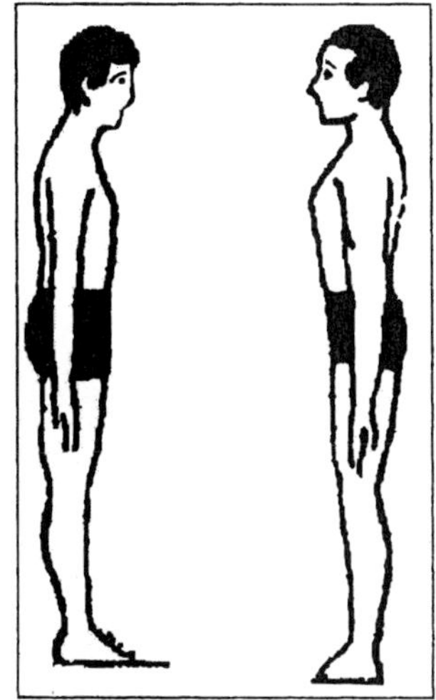

Our answer would be "Undoubtedly". You can set right your posture by effort and continuous practice. The older the habit of keeping the different parts of your body in a wrong position, greater will be the effort needed to get rid of it.

So it means that our posture becomes wrong due to our carelessness or ignorace. But if we exercise a check on it and strive to practise the correct posture, the wrong posture can be set right.

Several people, on the suggestions of their friends, walk with a stiff head or a protruded chest and think that they are following the correct posture. But they are mistaken. The posture does not become correct by making any part of our body stiff. For this we require systematic movements and regular practice. Tension is aroused in our body, when we make it or any of its part stiff artificially. But if we maintain a natural posture, our muscles become elastic and strong. The normal posture keeps our body and its parts healthy and dynamic.

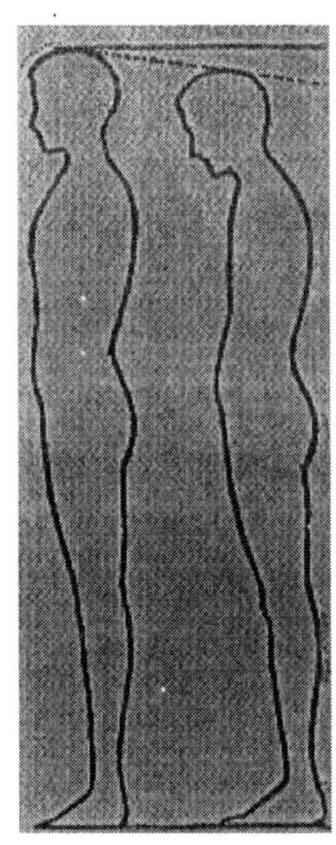

Why is correct posture essential?

Our posture is directly related to the activities of the internal parts of our body. Wrong posture hinders the right functions of heart, lungs and circulation of blood. The curves in the spine, fallen shoulders and drooping head do not allow the heart and lungs to function properly.

You can very well realise that if the heart and the lungs do not function properly, what will be the consequences thereof. You are thinking correctly. If the blood circulation is not proper our body and its parts become weak. There is pain in certain parts of the body, while stiffness is found in others. The man becomes tired and his hands and feet become benumbed. The cumulative effect of all these will be that your posture will become all the more defective. Consequently your stature will become still shorter.

Examine your posture yourself by standing before a mirror, or let one of your friends examine it. Thereafter, start improving the position of those parts of your body which have become defective.

But here you should keep one thing in mind. Suppose you have developed the habit of walking with your head bent. To remove the wrong position of your head, you should hold it erect. But do not put all pressure on one part of your body alone. While practising the correct position. of other parts of your body, the exercise of the head should also be done. Only then you will get good results. On the contrary, if you take more work from one part of your body, or a group of muscles, you will find that you will feel much more tired and the good results which you expect will be totally absent. On the other hand, you will have to endure its bad effects.

Follow the programme of improving your posture separately, but adhere strictly to one maxim. In whatever condition you may be whether sitting, standing, walking or lying, remain erect. Always remember that you have to sit erect, you have to stand erect, you have to walk straight and you have to lie straight. Not only does your body become straight while you sit erect or stand erect, but your stature also looks tall, for your entire body gets an opportunity to expand.

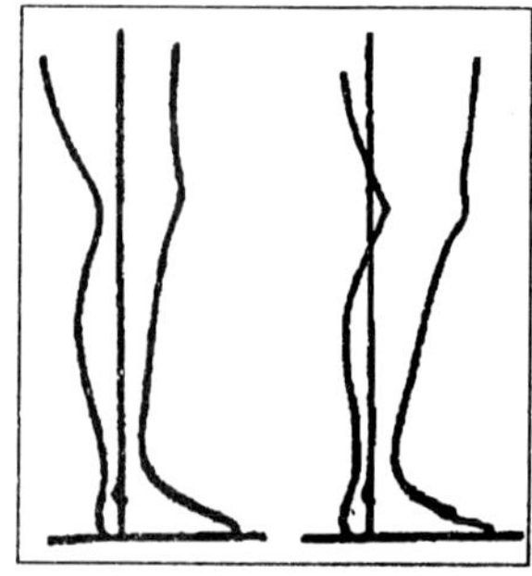

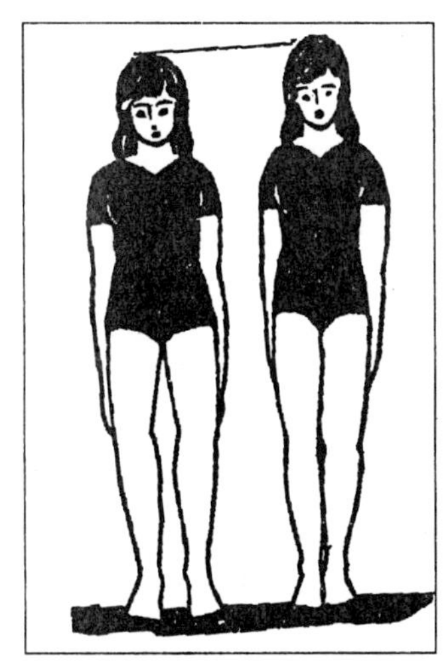

We would like to go a step further and say that when you try to stretch yourself fully, you go on expanding and within a short time your height begins to increase in inches and centimetres.

Right way of sitting, walking and sleeping

Sitting, walking and sleeping are different activities of human life. While sitting and walking fall under one group, sleeping comes under a different group. Our energy is spent in sitting and walking, while we regain the lost energy in sleep.

But you will be surprised to learn that many people make their bodies work even during sleep and do not regain the lost energy and alertness. Such people do not know the correct method of sitting and walking and spend a lot of excess energy in performing these activities. Consequently they feel tired every time. Hence they should learn the correct method of sitting, walking and sleeping.

The right way of sitting

(1) That is the proper way of sitting in which no part of the body is burdened unnecessarily.

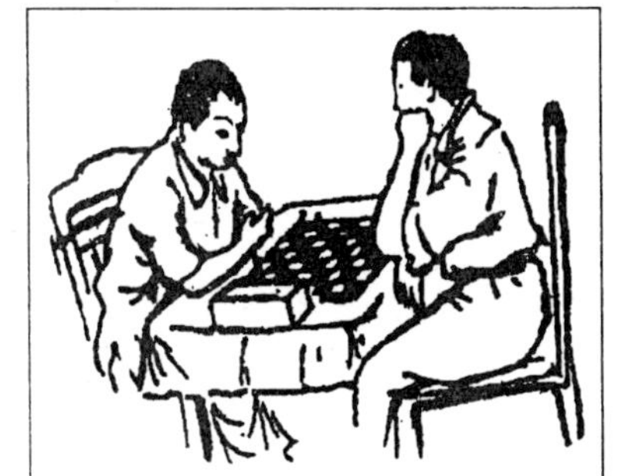

(2) While sitting, our back should get the right support.

(3) The height of the chair or stool should be such that undue pressure is not exerted on our thighs.

(4) There should be small chairs for children separately.
(5) The whole back should get support on the chair, right from the waist up to the shoulders. When you bend forward, the upper part of the body should come forward together as a whole and not only your neck or waist.
(6) When you feel tired, you may get up from the chair for a while. Do not become lazy and bend your shoulders or stomach in a wrong fashion, which would result in a wrong posture of your body.

The right way of walking

(1) The head should stand erect while you walk.
(2) The whole spine from neck to waist should remain erect, but undue strain should not be caused to any part thereof.

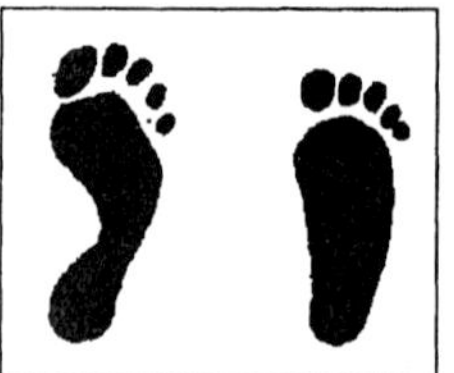

(3) The chest—should be duly stre-tched while walking.
(4) The hands should-not be kept inside the pockets, but the fists of the hands should be closed so that the arms can be moved freely.

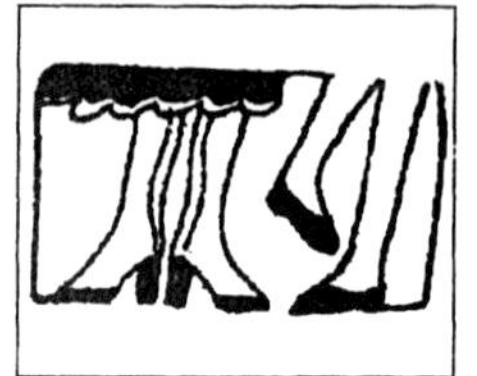

(5) It should also be kept in mind that while you walk, the different parts of your body should not lie in a loose and lethargic condition. Walk systematically. It should appear from your gait as if some victorious person is coming and dominating the nearby environment.

The right way of sleeping

While asleep our body tries to regain the energy lost during the day. Side by side the height of the body also increases during sleep. Hence we should bear in mind the following:

(1) The bed should be made of plywood.
(2) The bedding should be evenly spread on it.

(3) The pillow should be neither too thick nor too thin.

(4) The length and breadth of the bed should be of sucr dimension so that we can lie straight on it and both the sides, right as well as the left, easily.

(5) Two persons should never sleep together on one bed—children, too, should not be made to sleep with on the same bed. This creates a bad effect on development of the height of the body.

(6) There should certainly be a window in your bedroom. This would enable fresh air to come in and you can breathe freely.

These are very simple things no doubt, but they are of great importance. By acting on these advice, we can remove the hurdles in the way of increasing our height, while performing the various activities in our life such as sitting, walking, sleeping or waking.

Costumes—Costumes play an important role in showing one tall. If someone is wearing loose Kurta-payjama or dhoti-kurta, he will appear short. But if a man of same height is wearing a tight jeans & shirt will look taller.

If you wear cap on your head, you look a little tall. If you comb your hair in back direction or hair face sky, you look long, Ladies having Juda of their hair, look taller than the ladies of same height with one choti of their hair.

High heels are common among girls and ladies, which can add upto four inches to one's height. But beware, don't wear sharp edged heels; as this may cause fall and back-hip pain too.

Sikh's, who wear pagadi look taller than the persons of same height who do not wear it.

The persons (male-female) who are obese look shorts to those who are lean-thin, though of same height.

■

6

Effect of Rest Massage Sunshine and other Factors on Height

Rest, Sleep and Height

Most of us know the ways of working, but very few know the art of taking rest. They allow their muscles, brain and mind to function heavily during sleep. They keep on changing sides in bed and when they get up after eight or nine hours of sleep, they are not fresh for the work of the day.

Its main reason is that they do not know the technique of taking rest. It is very necessary to know the technique of taking rest, which we are describing here.

The aim of sleep is to give rest to our muscles and mind. You can give it in the following manner:

Lie down straight on a 'takhat' or on a bed made of ply wood. Have your bedding spread out evenly on it. Give rest to all the parts of your body. Take care to see that no part of your body is made to do any extra work. Resort slowly to deep breathing. Put out the light. Close your eyes and think of the 'dark night' in terms of any dark object. Remember God and bid farewell to all the activities of the day by saying "Good Night" to them. In no time you will fall asleep.

Our body gets fatigued by working throughout the day. The cells of the body get worn out and the stature is also somewhat reduced.

When we stretch our body to take rest, all the parts of our body get an opportunity to expand and develop. The pressure that is exerted on the backbone during the day time disappears. This affords an opportunity to the backbone to expand.

Taking rest and sleeping in this way increase the height of a person continuously.

If you are desirous of increasing your height you should sleep for nine to ten hours a day instead of eight while you are undergoing this course.

Always remember that 'sleep' is the main device of Complete Rest. Sufficient sound sleep acts as main tonic for increasing your height and strengthening your body. Take balanced diet and keep your digestion in order. This will enable you to have a sound sleep at night. Sleep during the day, breathe fresh air, walk in the morning as well as in the evening and take light exercise—all these will contribute to give rest to the body and the height will go on increasing.

It is the opinion of expert physicians of the world that we should keep our mind detached from the senses and sleep with our body fully stretched on a large-sized bed. Allow every part of your body to get rest and see its good result.

Massage and its effect on one's height

Massage is the scientific device to make the nerves healthy,' ensure proper blood circulation, and make the muscles flexible. We provide nourishment direct to the body through massage. As a result of massage, the parts of the body become active, fresh and efficient. The refuse is excreted quickly and the digestive system functions speedily. The pores of the body get opened. The stiffness caused in the muscles due to fatigue gets removed by massage. Due to its effect, the muscles become flexible, which results in their growth and development.

Massage is really the exercise of muscles. It is directly connected with the height of a person.

Massage has its own science. Here we will refer to it only in as much as it is related to the increase in one's height.

(1) *Massage of the back*—First of all lie down on the ground or on a hard bed supported on by your chest and stomach and let someone else massage your back. Get oil rubbed

on your back. Pay more attention to the backbone. Massage should be done from upwards to downwards followed by gentle patting. Pay special attention to both the sides of the back divided by the spine, and get both the sides massaged adequately by performing clockwise movements, stiff rubbing and patting. This leads to the increase in the length of the backbone which ultimately leads to the increase in the height of a person.

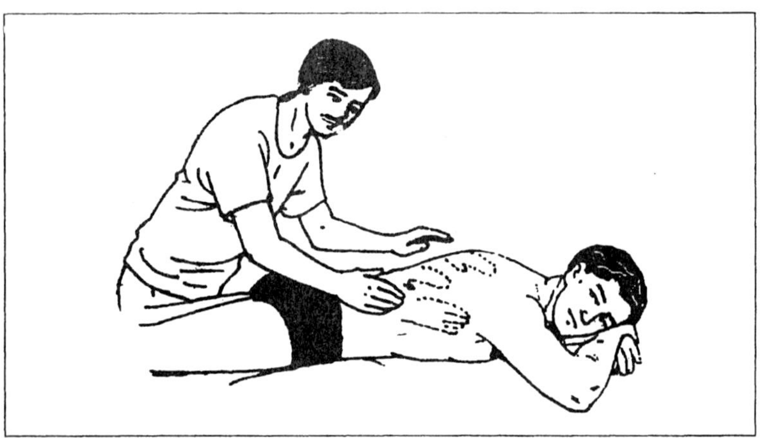

(2) *Massage of the neck, arms and legs*—Join both of your hands in the shape of a bangle. The massage should begin from the upper portion of the backbone. Get the neck, arms and legs massaged by the 'twist' technique. As a result of this the unwanted elements creating fatigue will not accumulate in your muscles and the blood circulation will become quicker. The result is that the different parts of the body are nourished. The massage of the neck (thyroid gland) increases the height of a person.

Massage the legs below the ankles and the soles of your feet as well.

(3) *Massage of waist, stomach and chest*—The massage of the waist and stomach should be done by a technique involving three processes: patting, rubbing and rolling.

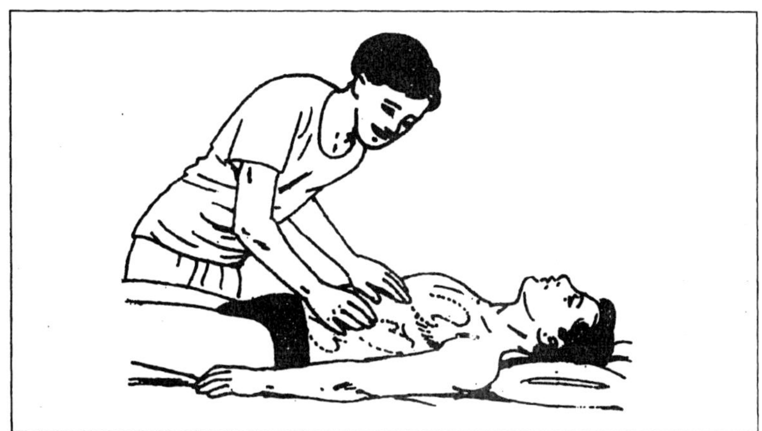

The stomach should be kept loose at the time of massage. Let the knees lie in a standing position on the legs. The stomach should be massaged only in the morning. This massage should be done with the help of oil. Massage can be done in a number of ways. Oil massage is the best. Besides, dry massage, powder massage, hot and cold massage can be done. People having greasy skin should resort to dry or powder massage.

The noon or evening massage can also be done with the help of powder or it can be dry.

Thus the growth of the body takes place when it is massaged properly, rubbed effectively and patted gently. The ladies should also massage their bodies like men and do it regularly. During pregnancy or the period of menses, the women should massage all the parts of their body except stomach and uterus.

Sunshine, fresh air and stature

Once a pair of twins was born in a hospital in Europe. At the time of birth both the children were of the same stature. The weight of one child was 3.34 kg while the other weighed 3.110 kg. The firsf child whose weight was 3.34 kg was kept in a place where there was no sunshine. The other child was kept in the open where there was plenty of sunshine. Both were given the same diet. They were medically examined after a month. The child who was getting sunshine and fresh air gained 3/4 kg in weight within one month. There was another surprise. The stature of the first child became shorter, while the other child grew in stature by three inches. This is the effect of sunshine and fresh air and reveals their importance.

Those who live on the peaks of mountains are found to be taller in comparison to their relatives, who live in valleys. Even in the same state it has been observed that those who work under the sun in the open fields are taller than those of their relations who live in the narrow lanes of big cities and those who work in factories. Have you ever thought as to how the offspring of the same parents are tall as well as short in stature? If one is tall, the other is short. How does the growth of one and the same person vary in different situations? You must have understood our meaning, the reasons are sunshine and fresh air.The famous english journalist, John Douglas says, "If some one would ask me to enumerate the three most valuable things of the world, I will say sunshine, fresh air and water." Vitamin D is present in the rays of the sun, and there is oxygen in fresh air. Water regulates the entire digestive system.

The sunshine is the essence of all physical powers. If human body is deprived of sunshine for some time, it becomes powerless and is surrounded by a number of diseases. Those people who work in dark rooms or underground rooms, find that their skin soon becomes pale and they suffer from anaemia.

We get light and heat from the sun. The old residents of Greece and Rome knew the importance of basking in the sun. They used to make use of the roofs of their houses to bask in the sun. Hippocrates, the father of medical sciences and Celsus were great exponents and supporters of the heat of the sun. They were of the opinion that those persons, who basked under the sun, developed great resistance against diseases. Celsus used to advise the patients suffering from nervous diseases to expose themselves to the sun.

The sun-bath should be taken in the morning sun. Put on an underwear and enjoy the rays of the sun without putting on any other clothing on the body. Slowly you will be perspiring. The circulation of the blood will increase in the whole body. The dormant or the dead cells of the body will revive. If oil massage is also done as suggested above, you can have a complete transformation of your body in a few days. Within a few days the height starts increasing.

Fresh Air

Enjoy fresh air along with the sun-bath both in the morning as well as in the evening while putting on light clothes. In the morning go to some garden and do the exercise of deep breathing. Enjoy as much oxygen as you can, inhale it and benefit your body thereby. You will find that you have become fresh. If you feel this freshness both in the morning as well as in the evening, do you know what it suggests? Yes, your freshness goes to prove that you are deriving the maximum advantage of the gifts of nature i.e., sunshine, air and water. If you are growing in harmony with nature, your body will naturally grow and develop.If a plant grows when it finds sufficient sunshine and water, why will not the human being grow when it also enjoys these gifts of nature?

■

Our Diet

Food is absolutely essential to keep a man alive. Three types of substances are derived from the food that we take. First those which act as a fuel for our body, second those which help us to recoup the damages done to our cells and tissues. The third substance helps in the improvement of our health. The diet which gives us all the three substances is called a 'balanced diet'.

Substances Found in our Diet

Our food mainly contains three elements: These are carbohydrates, protein and fat. Besides, several types of minerals and vitamins are also found in our food.

Here is a brief description of the substances found in our food:

Carbohydrate—Just as an engine requires fuel to run, similarly our body needs fuel, i.e. energy, which is derived from carbohydrates.

Carbohydrates are derived from starch and sugar in our food. Starch is derived from wheat, rice, barely, maize, pulses and potato. Sugar is derived from 'gur', glucose and sugar itself.

Protein—It is found in pulses, meat, fish, eggs, milk and curd. It is very necessary for the growth of our body and increase in our height. Since the body of a child grows faster, it requires more protein than what is needed for an adult.

Fats—Fats are found in oil, ghee, fish, eggs and milk. Fats give more energy to our body than the carbohydrates. We need more fats in cold weather to keep our bodies warm.

Minerals—Our body needs several types of minerals. It would not be relevant here to dwell upon them in detail. It would be sufficient to mention their names. For example, calcium, phosphorus, iron, bronze, sulphur, sodium, potassium, magnesium and chlorine. Of these the first three, calcium, phosphorus and iron are essential for the development of the body, for the increase in height and for making the bones strong. Iron is necessary for the formation and growth of red blood corpuscles. These minerals are found in milk, butter, meat, eggs and green vegetables. (Those desirous of increasing their heights should take these three according to a fixed schedule.)

Vitamins—They were discovered arourd 1890 by the scientists on the basis of their research. Vitamins are found in fruits, grains and vegetables, but some of the vitamins are destroyed or reduced in quantity when the food is cooked. Hence these days vitamins are also available in the market in the form of tablets, capsules and syrup. The use and intake of vitamins is necessary to maintain the strength and the working capacity of the body. Certain diseases are also treated by the use of vitamins— where disease is the outcome of deficiency of vitamins.

Vitamins are of many kinds A, B, C, D and E. Brief details about them are given below:

Vitamin A—This vitamin is very essential for the development of the body and the increase in one's height. It is very necessary for the strength of our bones and teeth. The eyes also grow weak due to the deficiency of this vitamin. This vitamin also increases the resistance of human body towards disease. The children should get this vitamin in sufficient quantity, so that the development of their body may be proper and the growth of their bones and teeth may not be hampered.

Vitamin A is found in sufficient quantity in milk, butter, cheese, cod liver oil and yellow of the eggs. Carotene which is found in green vegetables, such as carrots, turnip, radish etc., creates vitamin A when it enters our body. Vitamin A is also found in sufficient quantity in the liver of animals and also in tomato.

Vitamin B—It is really a complex of 12 vitamins. It is also called B-Complex. This vitamin is found in seeds, pulses, cabbages, carrots, eggs, liver, green vegetables, milk, cheese etc. The deficiency of this vitamin gives rise to the disease called Beri Beri.

Vitamin C—This vitamin is found in greater quantity in fruits such as lemon, orange, mausami, amla and tomato. It is also found in leafy vegetables. This vitamin helps our growth to a large extent. The bones of such children, who do not get this vitamin in sufficient quantity, do not develop properly.

Vitarnin D—This vitamin makes the structure of our bones strong. It is found in the oil of shark fish, liver, milk, an yellow of the egg. Due to deficiency of this vitamin, one may suffer from the diseases of bones and trouble in legs, the legs of children bend due to its deficiency. Their Limbs and the trunk of the body bulges out. Due to deficiency of vitamin D in young age, the bones lack in and phosphorus which create a tendency in them to break.

Vitarnin E—This vitamin is found in oil of the sprouting milk, meat, eggs and the whole grains. This is very necessary for the maintenance of the sex-health.

One should eat a balanced diet which is necessary for over all development.

What should we eat and when should we eat?

People often enquire from doctors, as to what they should eat so that they may remain healthy. According to the renowned American, W.R.C. Laitshun, this question can be answered in words: "Balanced Diet." He further says that there are factors which govern our diet. First is the mental condition in which the food is taken, second is the condition of the joints of the person and his digestion and the third, which is least important, is the content of food which is taken.

If you excited, worried or angry, you will not be able to eat the most nutritive and delicious food. If your stomach is not empty or your bowels clean, you will not be able digest the food that you take.

How much to eat?

The scientists on the basis of their research have analysed the various calories in the different items and have succeeded in determining the quantity of coories in proportion to quantity of food item.

According to this the general worker requires 2,800 calories per day and the staying within the house require only 2,400 calories. who do physical work need more calories.

In the same way, a young man requires more calories than grown up adult.

The different items of our food be changed frequently so that all the items may be i in our diet. An individual's diet schedule is proposed as follows:

Breakfast—Seasonal fruits, dry fruits, butter and toasts, one egg and a glass of milk.

Lunch

(1) Flour of wheat or rice 250 grams
(2) Dal 60 grams
(3) Ghee 50 grams
(4) Leafy vegetables, vegetables, curd, salad and raw vegetable.

Dinner—It should be light. You should fix your menu according to your taste and economic condition.

You should take light and easily digestible food both the times. While taking your meals, your mental condition should not be surcharged with emotions or restlessness. You should take your meals in a peaceful environment and without making haste. This is the ideal way of taking meals.

The Diet of Children

Our suggestion in this regard is that the children should be given such a diet which will make their bones strong and also increase their height. To achieve this end, you should give them pulses, ghee, butter, milk and rice in sufficient quantity. If this may not be possible, you may give them some of the following items in their breakfast. These are eggs, fish, tomato, apples, grapes or almond.

At the time of lunch, you should give them the soup of boiled nourishing vegetables such as beans. On special occasions you may give them dry fruits such as dry resins almonds nd dates.

The menu of the food at night can be fixed according to their taste. The meals at night should be lighter than the one in the morning, so that it may easily be digested.

Out of the liquid diets, you may give the children barley water, ovaltine, coco, along with other fruit juices. These drinks should be taken an hour after the meals.

The parents who are desirous of developing the body of the child and increasing its height should give nourishing diet to their children. Some children do not like the pulses, rice and vegetables, but want to eat pastries, tasty and fried snacks and sweets. Some like only potato and others want to eat the food of their choice like 'rajmah' only.

The parents should not yield to the obstinacy of the children, in such a condition. On the contrary, they should be explained with love that when only one item of food is taken, some ingredients become excessive in body, which is harmful. When other items of food are not taken, the body becomes weak, which gives rise to a number of new diseases. We believe that the children will value your arguments and your job will become easy.

■

8

Adequate Diet for Adults

Both tall and strong and short and weak statured persons live in the same country, same state, or same village. Have you ever thought as to why is it so?

The fact is very simple. The first type of people live systematically, take proper and nourishing diet, and eat in a proper way. The people of the second type do not live systematically, and they do not take their meals in a proper way. They are ignorant of the principles of diet. They do not even know as to what they should eat and how much they should eat.

So far as the question of taking proper diet to increase your height and to make your body strong is concerned, you should try to include in your diet-protein, iodine, calcium, phosphorus and iron. Side by side, the vitamins A, B-complex, C and D etc., should also be taken.

Protein: You can have protein from pulses, meat, fish, eggs, milk and curd. Protein is also available in cashew-nut, almond-nut, groundnut, peas and beans. If more protein is needed, you may buy protein powder from the market, which can be taken with milk or water as convenient.

Iodine: You can have iodine from tomato, green peas, fish etc. Iodine is responsible for the proper development of the body. It also increases the height of a person. It is also essential for making the thyroid gland strong.

Calcium: If bones have not developed properly, calcium will be needed in sufficient quantity to make its deficiency good. If calcium is not, procured in sufficient quantity from one's diet, the bones themselves draw calcium from their own resources. First of all they draw calcium from the vertebral column and later from the pelvic bones. If the calcium deficiency is not made good in time, the stature of a person remains short. Due to calcium deficiency the vertebrae of the vertebral column become weak. Due to weight, they develop unnatural curves. As a result of this the height of a person is reduced by a few inches. Quite a number of people develop hunches of their back. Due to calcium deficiency several defects enter the human skeleton. Hence calcium should be given to a man from the very beginning so that his height may increase as desired.

The calcium is available in milk in its natural form, but how many people are there in our country who can afford milk for their children as well as for themselves, in sufficient quantity? So calcium tablets can be had for them from the market. Cheese and green vegetables are good sources of getting calcium.

Phosphorus: It is available in a good quantity in wheat, milk, meat, beans and fruits having kernel. It is an important factor in the development of the bones.

Iron: It is an important mineral. Good sources of iron are green vegetables, eggs, potato and meat. Grams (black) when fried in an iron frying pan, yield iron in sufficient quantity.

Vitamins

In previous chapter we have given you an introductory knowledge of vitamins. They should be taken according to one's requirement for the development of the body, strengthening of the bones and for improving the eyesight. The vitamins A, B-complex, C and D should be taken according to the need of a person. For this a good doctor or a physician should be consulted so that he may recommend vitamin tablets, which should be taken regularly.

We are indicating below in brief the conditions in which vitamins become absolutely essential:

Vitamin A:

(i) For developing the body and increasing one's height.

(ii) To improve one's eyesight.

Vitamin B (Complex):

B_1—To get rid of Beri-Beri.

B_2—To treat the skin diseases.

B_{12}—To treat patients suffering from blood deficiency.

Vitamin C:

(i) To treat cases of scurvy.

(ii) To treat ascorbic deficiency.

Vitamin D:

To make the bones strong and ensure their proper growth.

■

9

Essential Food Nutrients—Necessary to Gain Height

All foods are rich in various nutrients, as no single food item is an all-contained item that can give essential nutrients to a person to meet his daily requirements thereof. In order to have balanced diet, certain vegetables, fruits, cereals, dairy products, poultry products are required to be blended or not taken in isolation, except when a particular situation demands. Following nutrients are said to be essential ingredients of a balanced diet:-

(i) Carbohydrates	(Sugar, wheat, grains, jaggery etc.)
(ii) Proteins	(Fish, grains, soyabeans, cheese, etc.)
(iii) Fats	(Saturated and unsaturated fats as butter clarified butter, vegetable oils)
(iv) Vitamins	(A, B complex, C, D, E, K)
(v) Calcium	(Milk)
(vi) Minerals	(Iron, phosphorus, manganese, potassium, etc.)
(vii) Dietary Fibre	Apples, Dried beans, Carrots, etc.

Carbohydrates: These are components of oxygen, hydrogen and carbon. They provide energy and heat to our body. Sugar and starch are well known sources of energy and both of which exist in green plants. Starch causes accumulation of fat in the body and it is difficult to digest, thus straining the liver. Lack of carbohydrates causes weakness, run-down condition and restlessness in the body, whereas its excess causes fatness (obesity). Liver retains them in the form of glycogen which is released by it, as soon as body requires it to sustain energy. Excessive release of glycogen into blood stream can cause rise in sugar levels of the blood and depressed or deficient supply can often result in low sugar percentage in the blood, both being forms of diabetes known as hyper and hypoglycemia respectively. A normal daily need of a person is 160 to 240 gms of carbohydrate which, often, is liable to vary depending on health status of a person.

Proteins: Proteins are required for proper development of our body and the word protein means' first in importance'. They are conglomerates of phosphorus, sulphur, carbon, oxygen, nitrogen, etc. and deficient supply of proteins to the body will compel the body to eat its own muscles so that all vital organs do continue to function in a normal way. Main function of proteins is to grow, repair and maintain organs and tissues of the body. In order to facilitate assimilation of proteins, the body releases amino acids which are more than 70 in numbers. Enzymes break the proteins into amino acids which, in turn, help protein to get absorbed into the blood stream. Out of 70 amino acids, 10 are considered essential for the purpose and such essential amino acids are known as high quality proteins. Chief sources of proteins are eggs, milk, soyabeans, almonds, nuts, fish and meats. Certain pulses, seeds, cereals, peas also contain protein but in a limited quantity, though their proteins also shell out good quality of protein. Pulses augment short supply of protein received from cereals. Hence, to get an added advantage, cereals, should always be taken with pulses.

Our skin, muscles, hormones and enzymes are composed of amino acids. Since their requirements are of permanent nature, so is the need for constant supply of proteins. In the absence or short supply of proteins to the body, one is liable to feel tired and weak, whereas their excess supply will vitiate our blood, as also let them rot in our intestines.

Daily requirement of protein of a person should be one gm per kg of body weight but it may be ensured that quality of protein is not inferior or substandard. For vegetarians, soyabeans are capable of giving almost double the amount of protein which an equal amount of fish can give. Is their any other bargain, in this respect, cheaper?

Fats: Fats discharge the function of lubricating the body, apart from being a concentrated source of energy and providing essential fatty acids for the aforesaid purpose. Our body's fat requirement is met from oils, pure fats. Apart from that some oil seeds, nuts, soyabean also supply fats. Pulses and cereals have meagre percentage of fats. It is a myth and a misplaced conception to totally eliminate oils from our diet. In fact, fats should form an essential part of our diet, as overuse is as dangerous and risky as total lack there of.

All oils and fatty acids have 3 types of fatty acids such as saturated (which are causatives of high rise of cholesterol in blood, if taken in excess), polysaturated acids do not raise cholesterol levels whereas monosaturated acids lower the level of cholesterol. Hydrogenated vanaspati oils are rich in saturated fatty acids and it also matters as to how and in what way they have been processed. Following table will clearly indicate the concentration of approximated quantity (percentage) in each variety of oil derived from various derivatives.

Oil	**%age of saturated fatty acids**	**% age of mono unsaturated fatty acids**	**% age of poly unsaturated fatty acids**
Butter oil	65	31	4
Coconut oil	91	6	3
Corn oil	13	26	61
Cotton Seed oil	28	19	53
Lard	43	45	12
Olive oil	14	77	9
Palm oil	53	37	10
Peanut oil	18	49	33
Sesame oil	16	41	43
Soyabean oil	16	24	60
Sunflower oil	11	22	67
Safflower oil	11	12	77

For a normal adult daily consumption of fat, from 25-35 gms, seems to be in order. Persons, doing hard and strenuous work, would require higher quantity of fat which should mainly be had from poly unsaturated fats., preferably vegetables. Heat generated by fats is almost double the amount of energy generated by carbohydrates, when process of oxidation takes place in the body. This energy is converted into body-heat and muscular work. Patients, who suffer from heart ailments, arteriosclerosis, high blood pressure or any other like disorder, should avoid saturated fats and substitute them with poly unsaturated fats. They should also avoid lard, palm oil, cream, butter instead they should lay stress on the use of skimmed milk and its bi-products.

Vitamins: Vitamins are essential ingredients of food. They assist carbohydrates, fats, proteins and other nutrients to promote various chemical processes, increase energy, replace and build cells. For maintaining good health, vitamins serve as protective foods. Following vitamins have, so far, been isolated.

Vitamin A: Its deficiency results in lack of appetite, night blindness, retarded growth, unhealthy skin, dental loss, depleted vitality and general growth. Its natural sources are fruits, vegetables, egg yolk. milk and its products, liver oil and liver of animals. In normal health one requires 5000 I.V. daily but in pregnancy and for lactating (nursing) mothers 8000 I.U. will do because its deficiency can lead to deficiency in milk secretion.

Vitamin B-I (Thiamine): Thiamine deficiency leads to depressed mental states, nervous irritation, weight loss, tickling sensation in the soles. It is of paramount importance for functions of muscles, nervous system, digestion, for promoting utilization of carbohydrates. Its daily normal requirement is 1.25 mg. It is derived from natural sources like pea-nuts, oat-meal, milk, rice husk, brewer's yeast, meat, liver etc.

Vitamin B-2 (Riboflavin): It promotes growth and general health, is useful for fine conditions of skin and eyes, helps body cells in using oxygen for release of energy from food and its deficiency may result in cracking of lip-corners and burning/itching of eyes. Its natural sources are milk and its products, whole grains, meat, liver and various foods. Its daily requirement, for a normal person, is 150 mg.

Vitamin B-6 (Pyridoxine): Its presence in essential in adding assimilation of proteins and fats, in blood building for normal functioning of brain, muscles and nervous system but its deficiency often results in disorders of nervous system, loss of hair, skin eruptions, loss of muscular control etc., Milk, banana, raisins, molasses, wheat germ, brain, brewers yeast, kidney, liver, fish, eggs, meats are natural sources of vitamin B-6. Its daily requirement is 2.0 mg.

Vitamin B-12 (Cobalamin): It helps is promoting growth of children, helps as a general tonic for the aged persons, in regenerating and forming R.B.C.s (Red Blood Corpuscles), nerve tissue and also in utilisation of carbohydrates, fats and proteins. Its deficiency often leads to lack of proper growth, inflammation of tongue (though quite occasional), fatigue and anaemia. Its natural sources are eggs, liver, meats, milk products, etc. Its daily requirement is 6.0 mgm daily, in normal course.

Vitamin B-5 (Pantothenic acid): Deficiency of this vitamin is often not found but, when it occurs, it may cause dizzy spells and disturbance in digestion. It is considered necessary for synthesis of antibiotics, nervous and digestive system. Its natural sources are brain, whole wheat, brewer's yeast, molasses, peas, kidney, liver etc. Said to blacken hair (not medically proved) For daily requirement 10 mg would suffice.

Vitamin-C (Ascorbic Acid): It builds up general resistance of the body, enabling the latter to fight infection, apart from hastening heeling. It is essential for healthy bones, teeth and gums, maintains vigour and good health, in restricting coughs, colds and sneezing. Its deficiency can lead to anaemia, bleeding from piles, lack of general resistance, etc. All citrus fruits are its major sources as also amla, mango, lime, lemon, tomatoes, potatoes, peppers, spinach and other vegetables and fruits. If stored or cooked, it is liable to be destroyed. Its daily normal requirement is 60 mg but may be required more in case of smoking, incessant sneezing and coryza. It may have to be increased to 500 mg daily, depending on severity and gravity of the case.

Vitamin-D (Calciferol): It helps in the formation of bones and teeth for utilisation of phosphorus and calcium. Its deficiency leads to rickets in infants and children. In pregnancy puffiness and swelling of feet, etc. indicate its deficiency, caused by malabsorption of calcium. Ultraviolet rays help to convert cholesterol, present in the skin, to calciferol. Its natural sources are milk, milk products, oil of fish and liver. Excess of this vitamin may cause toxic effects. Its daily requirement, for a normal person, is 400 I.U. But far higher dosage is required in pregnancy. Should never be used without medical advice and care.

Vitamin -E (Tocopherol): It helps in prevention of undesirable blood clots, and promotes formation of new skin (in the women). Its deficiency can lead to early aging, muscular disorders, loss of reproductive capacity. Its natural sources are wheat germ, grain and its products, leaf and green vegetables, margarine, vegetable oils, liver, eggs and butter and its daily requirement is 30 I.U. if situation demands. As for its importance, only vitamin C can be given with it.

Vitamin-K (Menadione): It assists in maintaining clotting system of blood. But for this vitamin and its capability to prevent clotting in blood, even a simple injury could have lead to fatality. For healthy and efficient working of liver it has an important part to play. It is found in wheat, brain, wheat germ, tomatoes, cabbages, potatoes, spinach, liver and egg-yolk. Bacteria, present in the human intestines, produces this vitamin, hence it hardly needs to be supplemented, but its use and importance cannot be overlooked or denied.

Note: We have mentioned only very prominent and generally used vitamins. In addition, there are other vitamins like

Niacin, Folic acid, Biotin, Vitamin F, Vitamin P (Bioflavonoid), Vitamin B-15.

Best course is to extract vitamins from vegetables and fruits and tablets or tonics should be taken only when the body is unable to extract vitamins from natural foods. All vitamins, falling under B-Complex category, are water-soluble and, thus, are drained out by system. If too much of vitamins are taken continuously for longer periods, it may render our body incapable of drawing vitamins from natural foods.

Minerals

There are five basic (or gross) minerals for the body such as, calcium, phosphorus, potassium, sodium and magnesium and trace elements consist of iron, copper, iodine, chromium, zinc and manganese, besides selenium. In addition, cobalt, nickle, sulphur, fluorine and gases (like oxygen, carbon, hydrogen and nitrogen). All such elements play an important part in physical well-being of the body, enabling it to discharge its functions efficiently. Calcium is meant for bones, iron for blood-building, iodine for warding off goitre and manganese to reduce risk of cancer. Improper balance between chromium and manganese may lead to heart disorders. If zinc is deficient, it is likely to lead to sexual dysfunction, anorexia (loss of appetite) and alopecia (baldness or loss of hair from the head).

Due to lack or deficient supply of minerals to our system certain physical upsets can be discerned. A brief account of important minerals is given below.

Calcium: It helps to form and maintain teeth and bones, blood to clot, in regulating cardiac rhythm and helps normal contraction of muscles. Calcium provides endurance and vitality, modifies menstrual pains, fortifies nerves. It also dispels depressed moods, loss of sleep, allergies of various origins, irritability of temper. Calcium deficiency is common in aged persons, menopausal state, smokers, etc. For absorption of calcium vitamin C and D are required. Its natural sources are milk and its products, leafy and green vegetables, citrus fruits, pea-nuts, beans sunflower seeds, soybeans, pulses, etc. If calcium deficiency is not made up from the above and other sources, the body takes up calcium from a person's bones. Calcium in conjunction with magnesium, helps in maintaining well-being of cardiovascular system.

Phosphorus: It is required for normal structure of teeth and bones and also for changing food enzymes into energy. It helps in absorption of calcium but, if in excess, it can make calcium uptake difficult. Phosphorus deficiency manifests itself in the form of general debility, pain in bones and lowered appetite. It helps to excrete, promote nervine health, hasten the healing process, and does not let calcium escape from the site of injury. Fat rich diet and crystal sugar help to maintain proper phosphorus. Calcium balance, whereas excess of magnesium/iron can block storage of phosphorus. Important sources of phosphorus are milk and milk products, seeds, nuts, fish, egg, poultry, meet, bread and whole grain cereals, pulses, beans, etc. Its supply to bone is adversely affected if antacids are used. It should never be taken by anyone of one's own, except under medical advice.

Potassium: Life would not have been possible without potassium which is a key mineral. Whole body chemistry is liable to be disturbed if body were to take it from the cells. Its deficiency will create a craving in pregnant women to eat clay/chalk. Its deficiency can cause weakness in muscle, irregular heart-beats, and irritable temperament but, its excess can cause various heart irregularities. It is essential for maintaining normal functions of nerves, muscles, cardiac functions and enzyme reactions, apart from regulating and balancing body fluids. Advancing age demands potassium in greater quantity for getting over muscle fatigue, inability to relax, constipation, itching on skin, nausea and cramps in the muscles. If such symptoms surface even in younger persons, it indicates deficiency of potassium. Higher intake of potassium can lead walls of blood vessels free from calcium deposits. Apple cider vinegar is an excellent source of potassium which (TSP mix with a glass of water), if sipped slowly, will emulsify fat, reduce high blood pressure, may also improve joints mobility. It (potassium) does not let sodium raise the blood pressure. Potassium deficiency could easily be prevented by a cup of coffee or alcohol in moderate quantity. It will also modify symptoms arising out of diarrhoea, liver torpidity, sweating or excessive use of diuretics. Its usual sources are dates, wheat germ, potatoes, cabbage, peas, peanuts, dried powder of skimmed milk, seeds, fish and poultry but, above all, from apple cider vinegar. Its daily intake is about 275 gms daily. More intake of sodium will increase loss of potassium, from inside the body cells.

Manganese: It helps in proper utilisation of vitamins B and E by activating various enzymes. It helps to remove indigestion and fatigue, helps blood clotting process and also produces more milk in nursing mothers. Since it increases glucose tolerance, it is useful in diabetes also. Its excessive intake will badly affect absorption of iron. Though its deficiency is hardly found in human beings, it can be easily obtained from whole grain bran, seeds, nuts, shell-fish, organ meats and black tea.

Magnesium: It is found in each cell of human body. Imbalance between calcium magnesium ratio can affect nervous system. Through our body contains hardly 50gms of it but, even then, its importance cannot be denied or overlooked. It helps to metabolise vitamin E and calcium. Its low content may even cause cancer, apart from causing diabetes. Vitamin B-6 and magnesium are known to have reduced risks of gall-bladder and kidney stones. It is found in abundance in hard water and those who drink hard water are reported to have negligible number of heart attacks. Strenuous physical exercises account for its depletion, often resulting in weakness, muscular contraction. It can be obtained from pulses, grain cereals, green and leafy vegetables, sea-food, dairy products and cereals, apart from hard water, as mentioned above.

Sodium: It assists in maintaining water-balance, inside and outside cells of the body. If taken in excess, it can trigger up blood pressure, cancer of liver, congestive cardiac disorders, renal diseases, but its deficiency can result in oedema, cramps in muscles. It is lost from our body through sweat and urine. It is not easily obtained from the content of sodium found in foods, hence its deficiency is made up by common table salt (Sodium chloride). Its excessive intake is far more dangerous than its depletion which can be easily compensated from meats, processed food and sodium itself.

Zinc: Zinc performs lots of functions, either alone or in conjunction with other factors. It handles functioning of protein and carbohydrates and aids in normal functioning of tissues. Too much use of alcohol, food refining, low-protein diet, pregnancy, cold and diseases can cause its deficiency which,. in turn, can lead to retarded growth process, loss of appetite and taste, delayed healing of wounds, lack of sexual maturity and dysfunction of reproductive system. Intestines are equipped to dispose of extra quantity of zinc which the body does not require. As the age advances, zinc deficiency may occur. Zinc is found in plenty from processed cheese, brewer's east, nuts, seeds, brain, wheat germ, rice (brown in particular), spinach, cottage cheese, poultry eggs and sea food, whole grains. Flour of whole wheat and its products contain four times more zinc, as compared to white flour.

Apart from the aforesaid minerals there are others too, like lead, aluminium, cadmium and mercury which are heavy metals but are not so significant as the above mentioned ones.

Dietary Fibre

It is the component that makes the cell walls in the plants and is non-digestible, due to the fact that it cannot be broken down by body enzymes nor can it be absorbed by the body and, perhaps due to this very reason, it was thought to have no dietary value and, thus, discarded. But the said conception was wrong in so far as it implied that it had no mechanical properties, But reality was totally otherwise, as it has the capacity to trap water, to keep the faeces moistened, thus removing constipation. But for the dietary fibre, intestines would never have been able to expel faecal matter, thus reducing the risk of accumulation of toxic substances and inflammation in the intestines.

Barley, oats, legumes and fruits have rich soluble fibre content, whereas wheat and most other cereals and vegetables have more insoluble fibre in them. The former help to lower serum cholesterol level but raise good cholesterol HDL, but the latter relieve constipation and improve digestion.

To affect reduction in weight, high fibre diets are more useful, for it takes much longer to chew them, gives more satisfaction to the eater, requires expense of more energy, reduces appetite and are stomach-friendly as they provide sense of fullness, Fibre helps in formation of stool, renders it bulkier and softer. The more the bulk and softness, the easier it is for the intestines to expel them. That is why cabbage and carrots are a preferred choice for those who wish to remain free from costive bowels. Bed-ridden patients should not take high fibre diets. A high fat-diet is always a low-fibre diet and high fibre diet is always a low-fat diet and further. "A high fibre diet tends to lower the blood pressure of hypersensitive persons."

Cholesterol

It is a yellow-white, waxy element produced mostly in the liver, and is a master molecule that plays an important role in lives of all beings. It is like a building block that the body uses to make other elements in the body. It is essential for survival of human life. Cholesterol is part and parcel of muscles, fat tissues, brain and nerves and, if it is between 140-160 mg, it is said to be within normal limits in a normal healthy person. It is generated by diet and is active in metabolic processes of blood plasma, liver and intestines. Serum cholesterol level beyond 240 mg is high, below 240 mg and up to 200 mg tolerable, and from 160-200 mg is normal.

It is triggered and precipitated by risk factors, like high blood pressure, smoking, obesity, diabetes, disorder of circulation, sedentary life and lack of physical activity, heredity, more in male gender and aged persons- all these factors are held to cause fall in low HDL (High density lipoproteins). It is the LDL that is the chief factor (low density Lipoproteins) for causing calcareous and crustaceous deposits in the arteries which, in turn, block the passage of blood. Efforts should always be made to raise HDL through diet and thus, lower LDL level. LDL can be effectively lowered by soluble fibre obtained from sunflower seeds, pectin (found in apples and citrus fruits) and corn, in addition to niacin, chromium, magnesium, oat bran, dry beans, etc. (which are other sources to lower LDL and raise HDL).

Of all the contributory causes, saturated fats are the major sources for raising cholesterol levels in the blood. So, consumption of red meats, chicken, whole milk, dry fruit should be avoided. Lack of exercise, sedentary habits, gluttony, obesity are other causes, Let fruits and vegetables play an important role in dietary menus of each home.

■

10

Calories, Height-Weight and Essential Nutrients

Table of Calories Burn in Physical Activities

In the following table an effort has been made to spell out calories spent by an individual in relation to his/her physical activity (For all sexes age-groups).

Activity	Calories expended per hours
(i) Light Activity	**50-200 Calories's Group**
Lying down/sleeping	80
Sitting	100
Driving a Car	120
Household work	180
(ii) Moderate Activity	**200-300 Calories's Group**
Bicycling (8.25 kms)	210
Walking (4.25 kms)	210
Gardening	220
Canoeing (4.25 kms)	230
Golf	250
Lawn-Mowing (Power mover)	250
Lawn-Mowing (Hand Mover)	270
Bowling	270

Continued

(iii) Marked Activity	**300-400 Calories's Group**
Walking (6 kms)	300
Swimming (40 Mtrs.)	300
Rowing (4.25 kms)	300
Fencing	300
Badminton	350
Horse-Riding (Trotting)	350
Roller-Skating	350
Volley Ball	350
Square Dancing	350
Table-Tannis	360
(iv) Vigorous Activity	**Over 400 Calories's Group**
Ice-skating (16 kms)	400
Sawing or wood-chopping	400
Tennis	420
Hill-climbing	480
Skiing	490
Hand ball	600
Bicycling (21 kms)	600
Running (16 kms)	900

Table of Daily Calorie Requirements (during 24 hours)

Age Group	**Calorie Requirements**
upto 6 months	120 Calories per kg body weight
7-12 months	100 Calories per kg body weight
1-3 years	1200 Calories
4-6 years	1500 Calories
7-9 years	1800 Calories
10-12 years	2100 Calories
13-15 years (boys)	2500 Calories
13-15 years (girls)	2200 Calories

Continued

16-18 years (boys)	3000 Calories
16-18 years (girls)	2200 Calories
Men, doing light work	2200 Calories
Men, doing medium work	2800 Calories
Men, doing heavy work	3400 Calories
Women, doing light work	1900 Calories
Women, doing medium work	2200 Calories
Women, doing heavy work	2800 Calories

Note—Parameters, shown above, are merely indicative of general standards but calories for each person are required to be worked out on the basis of age, sex, amount of manual labour put in, health status, person's height, weight and climate of a place.

Daily Calorie According to Body Weight and Activity (Daily Calorie Requirement in Food)

(Per kg Body Weight)

Weight of a Person	Office Workers (Light Work)	Medium work	Hard Work
Under weight	35	40	45
Normal weight	30	35	40
Overweight	20	25	30

Note: For Athletes, sports persons, persons engaged in strenuous work, children in growth period, pregnant women and man with malnutrition, calorie requirement should be measured in relation to physical condition and the amount of calories expended or expected to be spent. Each case has, naturally, to be individualised because no two cases could be identical. Since weight also must commensurate with height of a person and, in keeping with requirements of these two factors, following table will give an idea as to whether a person's weight is in proportion to his height.

Table of Ideal Body Weight in Kgs. and Height in Cms

Height (in cms)	Age Groups 18-20	23-27 (Weight in Kgs)	28-32	33-37
150	45.5	47.0	48.3	49.4
152	46.2	47.8	49.7	50.4
154	47.1	48.7	50.3	51.4
156	48.0	49.7	51.4	52.6
158	49.5	50.8	52.5	53.7
160	50.0	52.0	53.7	54.9
162	51.2	53.2	54.9	56.1
164	52.4	54.4	56.2	57.2
166	53.7	55.7	57.6	59.0
168	55.1	57.2	59.9	60.0
170	56.5	58.7	60.6	62.2
172	58.2	60.2	62.1	63.9
174	59.5	61.7	63.7	65.6
176	61.0	63.3	65.3	67.3
178	62.5	64.9	67.0	69.0
180	64.1	66.5	68.7	70.7
182	65.7	68.1	70.4	72.4
184	67.3	69.7	72.1	74.1
186	68.9	71.4	73.8	75.8
188	70.5	73.1	75.6	77.8
190	72.1	74.8	77.4	79.6

Height (in cms)	Age Groups 38-42	43.47	48.52	Above 53 Years
150	49.8	50.1	50.3	50.5
152	50.8	51.1	51.3	51.5
154	51.9	52.2	52.4	52.1
156	53.0	53.3	53.6	53.7
158	54.1	54.4	54.7	54.9
160	55.3	55.7	56.0	56.3
162	56.6	57.0	57.4	57.7
164	58.0	58.5	58.9	59.2
166	59.5	60.0	60.4	60.8
168	61.1	61.6	62.0	62.4
170	62.8	63.2	63.7	64.1
172	64.5	65.0	65.5	65.9
174	66.2	66.7	67.3	67.7
176	67.9	68.4	69.1	69.5
178	69.6	70.2	70.9	71.3
180	71.3	72.0	72.9	73.2
182	73.0	73.8	74.5	75.1
184	74.8	75.6	76.3	77.0
186	76.6	77.4	78.1	78.9
188	78.4	79.2	79.9	80.8
190	80.2	81.0	81.7	82.7

Note: + 5% weight should be taken as normal weight or, to be precise, marginally high/average weight. But + 15-20% weight, over and above the ideal weight, should be considered as 'overweight' and the latter calls for a guarded and modified approach in tapering and slashing down calories but, care should be taken that calories are not reduced to such an extent that a person gets weaker and is not in a fit frame to discharge even his normal chores.

Table of Daily Average Requirement of Essential Nutrients

Vitamins Vitamin 'A'	Daily Requirement
(For Normal Person)	5000 I.U.
(For Pregnant Women)	8000 I.U.
B-1 (Thiamine)	1.25 mg
B-2 (Riboflavin)	1.50 mg
B-6 (Pyridoxine)	2.00 mg
B-12 (Cobalamin)	6.00 mg
Niacin (Nictoinamide)	20 mg
B-5 (Pentatonic Acid)	10 mg
Botanic and Folic acid	0.31 mg
Vitamin-C (Ascorbic Acid)	60 mg
Vitamin-D (Calciferol)	400 - I.U.
Vitamin-E (Tocopherol)	30 I.U.–400 I.U.
Vitamin-F	Not clear
Vitamin-K (depending on clotting condition)	S.O.S.
Vitamin-P (Bioflavonoid)	Not clear
Minerals and Trace Elements	
Calcium for growing children	500-800 mg
Calcium for Nursing/Lactating Mothers	1000-1400 mg
Calcium for Adults	400-500 mg
Chromium	1-2 mg
Copper	2 mg
Iron	12-15 mg
Iodine	01– .02 mg
Manganese	5 mg

Continued

Magnesium	200-400 mg
Phosphorus	1 mg
Potassium	1000-4000 mgm (1-4 gms)
Sodium	400-1500 mgm
Selenium	50-200 mgm
Zinc	10-15 mg

Note: The aforesaid details are based on daily requirements of a normal and healthy person and are, thus, general and not particular indications. Every case has different expenditure, health status/diseased conditions, age, sex, regional climate, availability of recommended food items, and capacity of a person to purchase. In short, all efforts should be made to derive energy from available natural sources, such as vegetables, sea-foods (including fish), grain cereals, natural water resources, animal foods & products (like milk, butter, clarified butter, cheese, whey etc.), poultry products. As far as possible, try to avoid branded and commercial products and medicines, tinned and exposed foods etc. Emphasis ought to be on quality of the food but never on the quantity.

■

11

Exercises for Increasing Height

Start 10 movements which you have to practise regularly every day in the morning. There should be no exception.

The Morning

Out of the ten movements, the first nine movements will take one minute each and the last movement will take three minutes. Normally a minute's rest is advised after every movement.

Take five minutes rest after performing the first five movements. Thus you have to finish this programme in a total period of 25 minutes.

Do this exercise on all the seven days of the week. The ladies should give a gap of three days during the period of their menstruation. (or till such time the blood discharge continues.) The exercise should be started again after the period of menses is over. Of course, they can perform such exercises even during the period of menses, which will not cause harm to their sexglands.

The Mid-day

The men and women, who perform desk work during the day and housewives who do sewing work in the day, should practise the movements related to making their bodies tall and straight.

The Evening

Iri the evening one should go to the garden and do the exercise connected with catching the ball and hanging on the rod. One or two movements related to increasing the height in a play-way fashion should be done every day.

If these movements are practised continuously for three months, the height can increase by several inches.

How to perform this programme of movements?

You can derive extraordinary benefit from this programme only when you do not give any exception. Hence perform these exercises regularly and do not give any gap. Note down briefly the movements performed by you in your diary.

But if, per chance, an exception occurs you should not lose courage. Note down the date when a gap occurs, in your diary and continue your practice thereafter. Do this week by week and month by month.

The Morning

The course for the morning is scheduled for 25 minutes, that of the mid-day for 5 minutes and the programme for the evening is meant for 15 minutes. Thus you have to spend only forty-five minutes in twenty-four hours to derive the desired results from our programme entitled "Increase Your Height and Improve Your Posture."

The ten movements to be performed in the morning have been divided into 25 minutes. Keep a stop-watch with you and divide your time accordingly. Allot one minute to each movement. In the beginning you can take the help of some other person to give you the relevant cautions, such as, 'STOP' and 'START'. Later on, you will yourself get the idea of time and you will be able to perform these movements freely and efficiently.

First Movement

Running on the spot

This movement creates warmth in the body. It is proper to begin the programme of exercises with this movement.

Consequently, the blood-circulation increases in the whole body and all the parts of the body become alert. This movement acts 'I as an introduction to the movements that follow. Whether you are young or old, you can perform this movement without the least difficulty.

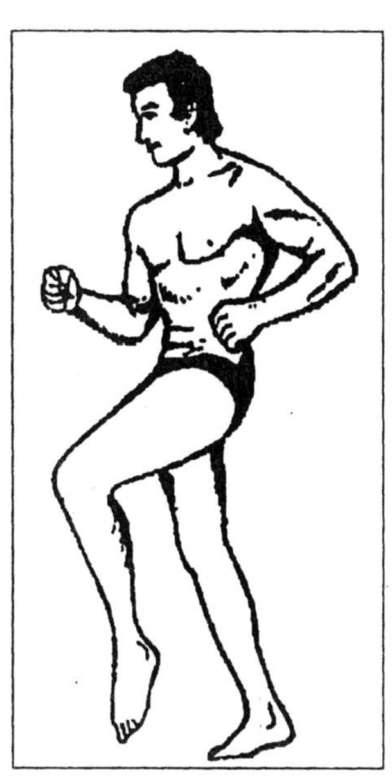

Note: Those patients who suffer from heart-trouble should not perform this movement.

Technique

Close your fists and move one leg after another, by turns. 'Increase your speed slowly. Keep your hands and feet moving as much as possible, but in a natural form. Perform as many movements as you can easily do.

Time: One minute.

Second Movement

Touching a mark on the wall

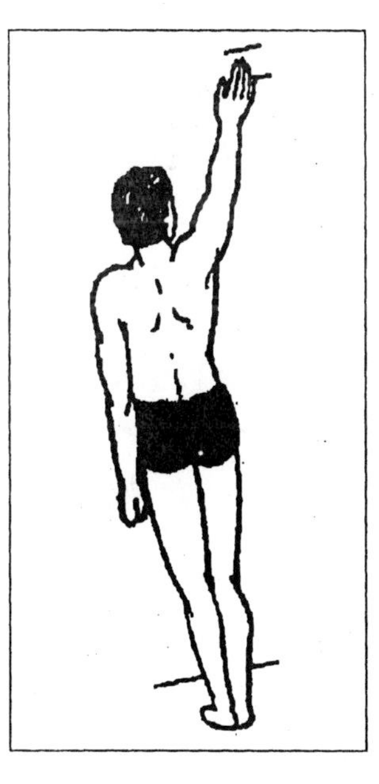

Stand erect close to the wall by joining both the legs and calves. Raise your right hand and touch the wall. Get a mark made on the wall by some one, within the reach of your hand.

Then get him make four or six marks on the wall with dark ink, each at a distance of half an inch from the previous one. Get these marks numbered.

Now stand in the same fashion as indicated before and try to touch as many marks on the wall as you possibly can. See how many marks you can touch. Repeat this exercise every day. You will find that your height is increasing.

Repeat this exercise daily, twice with both the hands, i.e., once in 15 seconds.

Time: One minute.

Third Movement

(i) Stretch your legs together on the ground. Both the ankles should be kept together. Sit erect making an angle of 90°.

(ii) Now take the upper portion of your body towards the back and make an angle of 120 degrees. Stay for a while in this position.

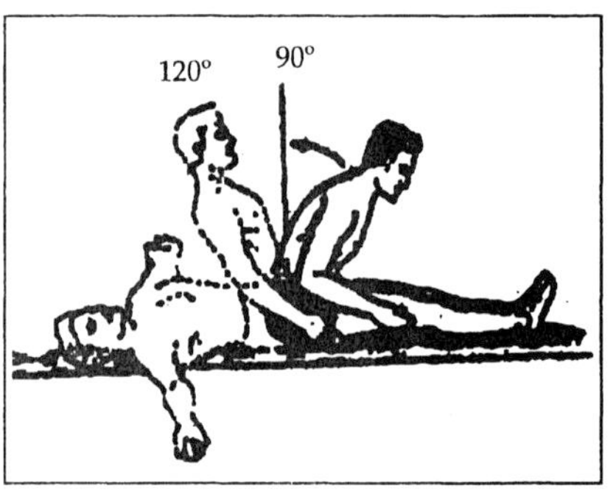

(iii) Gradually take your body (upper portion) backwards and lie down on the ground. Stretch both of your hands towards the right and the left part of your body.

Let the muscles be left loose now and practise deep breathing.

Repeat this four times.

Time: One minute, 15 seconds for each turn.

Fourth Movement

Exercise of the waist

Lie down supported on the back of your body.

(i) Close up the fingers of both the hands together in the shape of a paw. Gradually bend the right leg at the knee and holding the knee with the paw bend it towards your chest. Take care to see that the lower part of the waist remains firmly on the ground and the left leg also lies straight.

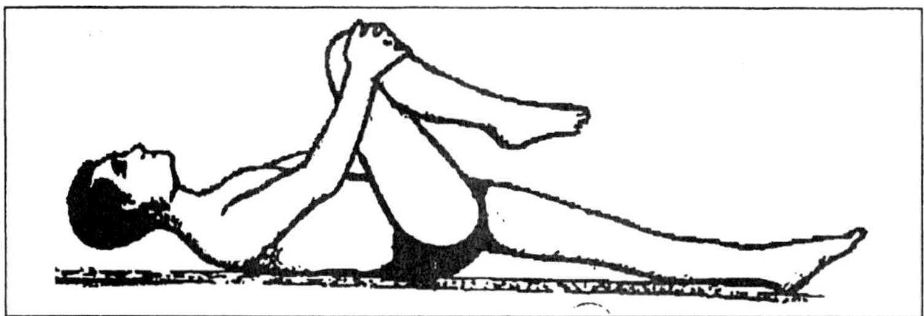

(ii) Now repeat this exercise with the left leg. In that case the right leg will lie straight on the ground.

(iii) Now practise this exercise with both the knees. You should see that the lower part of the waist remains firmly on the ground. Practise the three exercises for ten seconds each. Repeat the whole exercises twice.

Time: One minute.

Fifth Movement

To make the shoulders and the body flexible

(i) Stand erect and keep both the legs at a distance of one foot from each other. The chest should bulge out, neck should remain erect and both the arms should be kept downwards like a perpendicular.

(ii) Now raise your arms upwards.

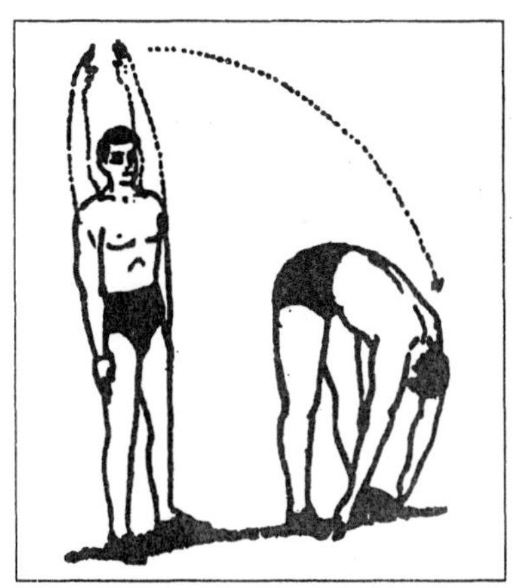

(iii) Next, bend downwards and touch your feet with your hands.

Repeat this movement four times within a minute, i.e., one movement should be performed within 15 seconds.

Note: Heart-patients should not perform this exercise. Time: One minute.

Five movements for women

First Movement

Expanding the chest

This movement expands the chest, the shoulders become strong, the posture improves, physical tension disappears and there is proper circulation of blood in the head and the brain.

Technique

(1) Stand erect in an easy and comfortable position. Raise your arms and keep the palms of both of your hands close to your chest facing each other.

(2) Take your hand as much behind your back as possible. Close your fists and expand your chest.

(3) Take your close fisted hands as much upward towards your back as you possibly can and bend your backbone upto your waist. Keep your head forward as much as you

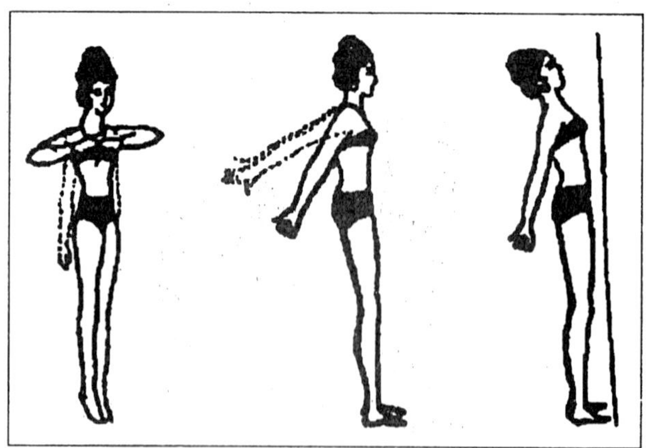

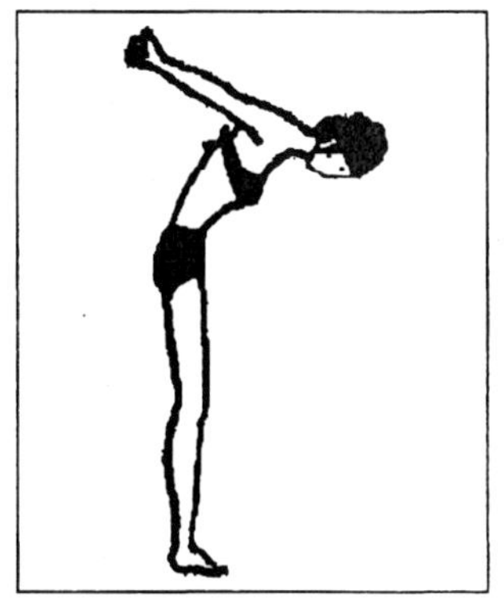

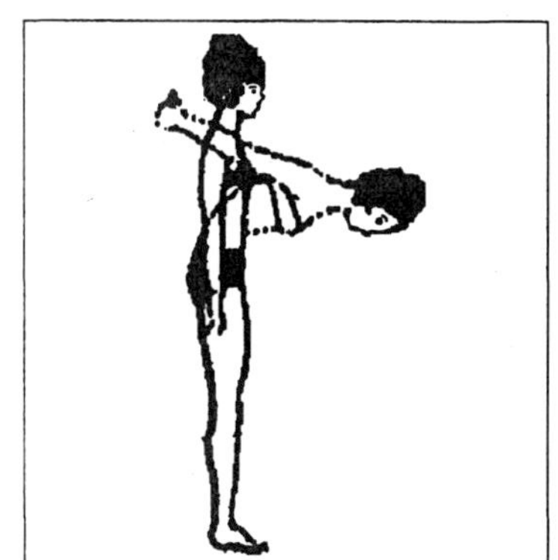

can easily do, but take care to see that the hands remain in the back.

(4) Open the fists gradually and stand erect. Repeat it for one minute.

Second Movement

Jump and catch the ball

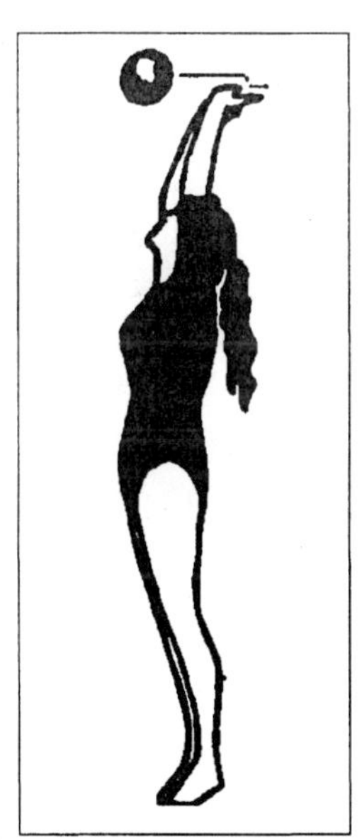

Take a ball and throw it over your head, a little bit jump and try to catch the ball. Try to catch the ball yourself by throwing it in upper directions so that in different portion of the legs, arms and back move freely.

You can do this exercise even in the evening.

Time: One minute.

Third Movement

(i) Sit stretching your legs on the ground and keep your face in the front. Let the left leg be pressed below and keep the right hand on the left.

(ii) Stretch the right leg in a straight position.

Now, do the exercise with the left leg and change the position of your body accordingly.

Time: One minute.

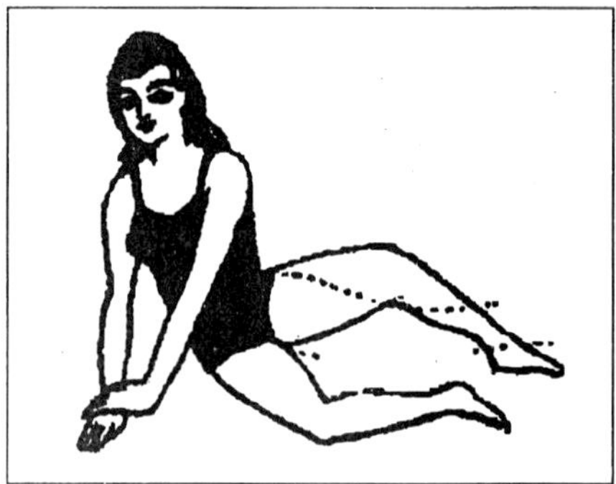

Fourth Movement

Exercise of the waist

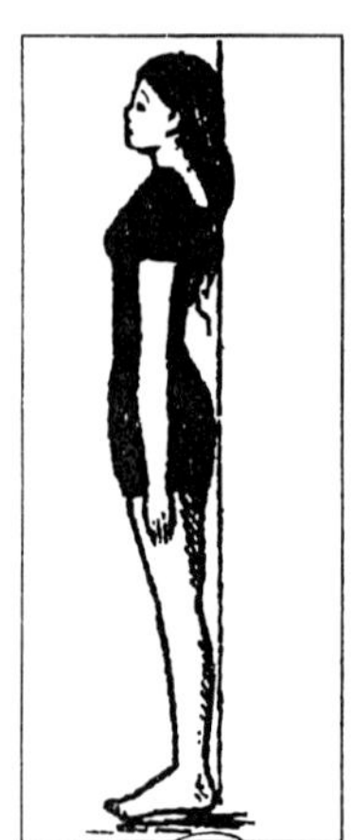

Stand by the wall. Take care to see that all the parts of your body touch the wall: heels, hips, back and head. Take a deep breath and try to shrink your hips. Try to touch the wall with the hind portion of the waist. This part of the waist will touch the wall only when you will breathe deeply inside. Remember that while you breathe deeply, the stomach should shrink inside. Now, take rest by standing' at ease'. Complete the exercise within one minute.

Fifth Movement

To make the arms and legs flexible

(i) Stand erect. Give some rest to your right hand and right leg.

(ii) Gradually lift your right arm straight upwards. See that your head remains erect.

(iii) Bend your left leg gradually backwards and hold your leg with your left hand. Keep your right arm upwards as before."

(iv) Bend your right hand and head a little behind and pull up your left leg a little over your back.

(v) Take rest for a while Repeat this exercise with the right leg, by turning in the opposite direction.

Time: One minute.

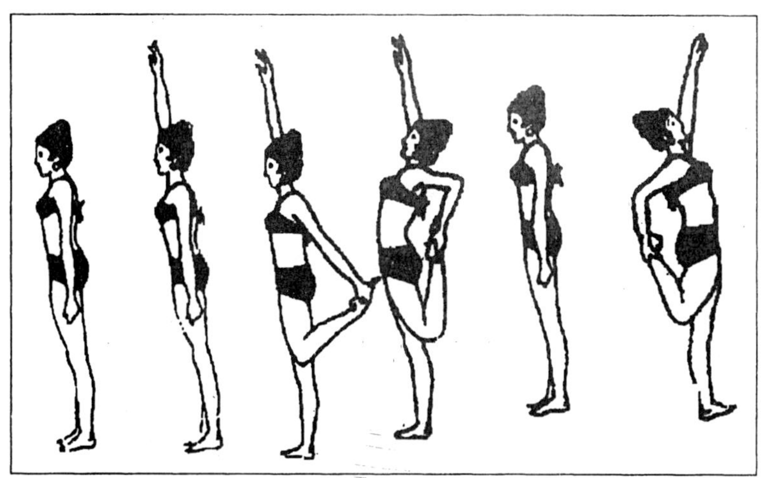

Five movements common to both men and women

Stretching the Vertebral Column

(1) Lie down straight on your back. Leave the body loose and breathe.

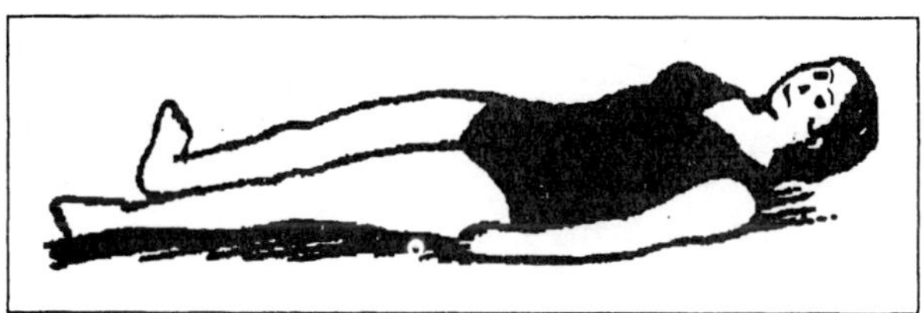

Now take deep breath. Hold your breath for a while and raise your shoulders upwards. Turn your legs in such a way that both the knee-caps face each other and toe on one foot touches the toe of the other.

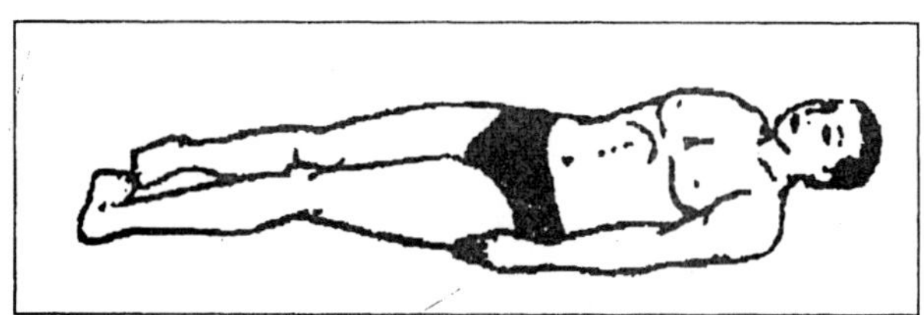

Release the breath slowly and bring your arms at their own place. Keep the knee-caps in their natural position. Complete this exercise within 15 seconds.

(2) Now, lie straight on your back as you did in the first position. Breathe and let your body lie loose. Hold your breath for a while, as you did in the previous exercise, and raise your shoulders towards your head. Bend your legs in a direction opposite to the previous one. Turn your legs in such a way that the joints of the ankle touch the ground. This exercise should also be done by holding your breath. The breath should be released only after you have reached the final stage of exercise.

Perform both of these exercises twice by turn and not more. After performing this exercise, leave the body loose in a state of rest for some time.

Time: One minute.

Movements while lying supported on the stomach

(1) Lie down on the ground taking the support of the stomach. Let your arms rest fully on the ground on both the sides of your body. Your chin should also touch the ground. Bend your legs at the knees and try to stretch the soles of your feet towards your back.

(2) Now hold both of your feet with both of your hands. Exerting pressure on them, try to raise your chin as much above the ground as you can. Leaving the legs apart, and remain lying on the ground with the support of the stomach, for a few moments. In this condition only the stomach touches the ground and the chest and the thighs are raised above the ground.

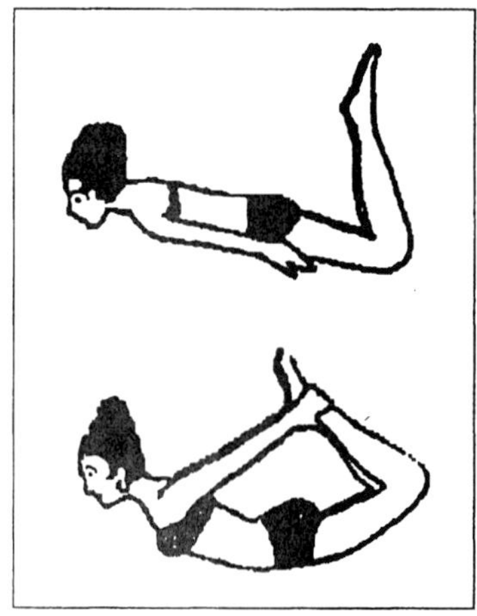

Now revert to the first position. Let the arms lie straight on both sides of your body. The whole body from chin to the knees will lie on the ground supported on the stomach. The legs will be bent upwards from the knees.

Gradually straighten your legs. Breathe deeply and change the sides.

Repeat this exercise by turns. Each turn will take 16 seconds. Do it twice.

Time: One minute.

Swinging on the rope

Fasten a rope in the iron bangle (kundi) in the ceiling. Tie a small wooden rod at the other end of the rope, so that you can swing by holding it in both of your hands. Now, hold it and swing. As far as possible, keep your mouth closed while swinging. Stop in between and take rest. Swing again. Stop swinging when you feel tired.

Note: (1) The rope can also be tied to a high door or to a thick branch of a tree.

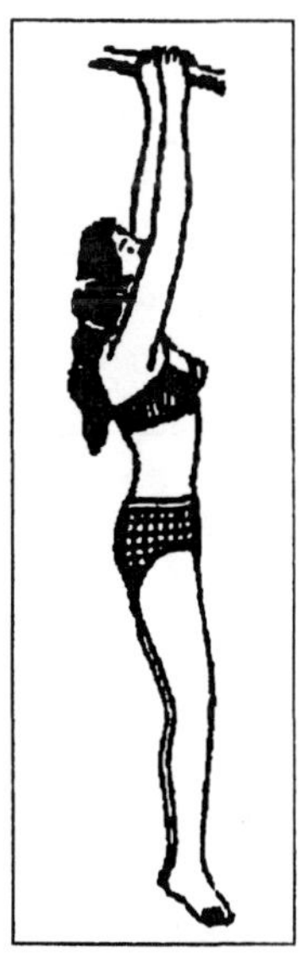

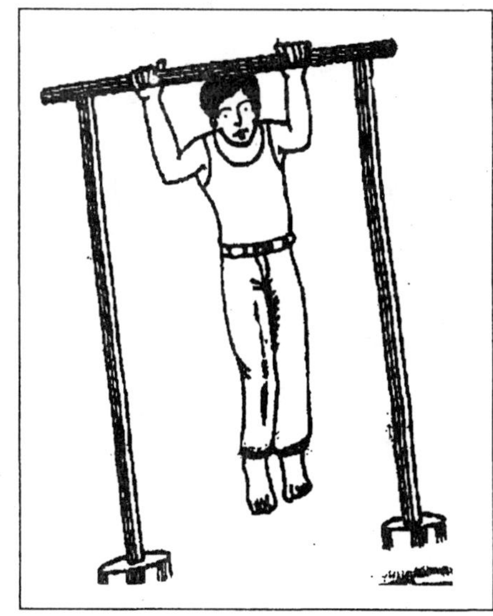

(2) Weak ladies and gents can sit in a swing and perform these movements easily.

Time: The same one minute.

Swinging on the rod

You can swing on the iron rod fixed to a stand on the ground. The rod should certainly be at least at a height of one foot from the reach of both of your hands.

While swinging on the rod, move your feet high with a force and give a push. This will bring speed in your swinging. If your breathing becomes fast and you start perspiring, stop for a while and take rest. Swing again after the moments of rest are over.

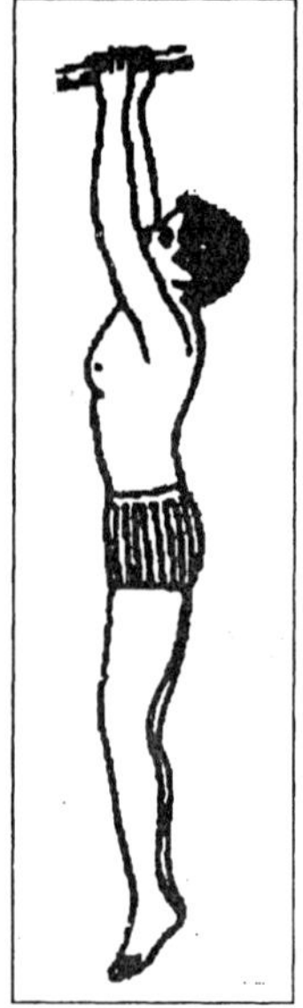

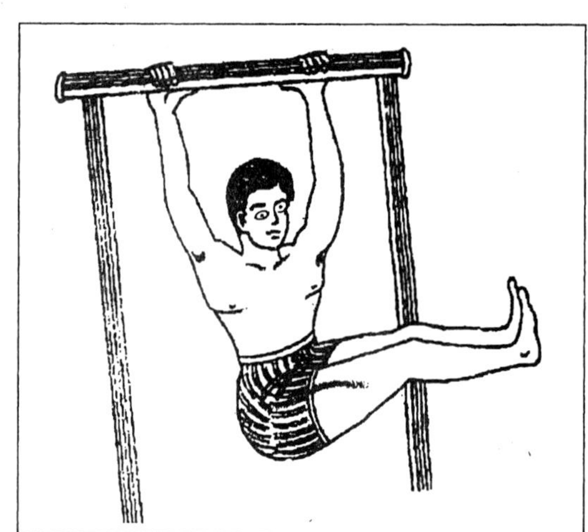

Even ladies can swing in this way, if they are in a normal condition. Fat persons and those suffering from heart disease should not perform this movement.

Time: One minute.

Kick Exercise-Reverse

Stand behind a chair. Hold the upper part of the chair with both of your hands and bend forward. Raise the right leg

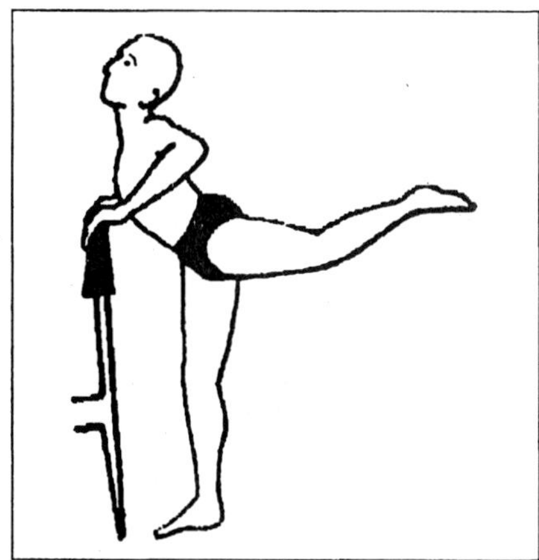

slowly towards the back, as much as you can. Take care to see that the entire leg is lifted in the position of a straight line, without bending at the knee. Remain in this position for 5 seconds. Breathe comfortably. While performing this exercise keep your chin upwards.

Repeat this exercise with the left leg.

The movements of both the legs should be performed four times.

Time: One minute.

The posture of rest (Time: One minute)

Concentrate your attention on giving rest to each muscle of the different parts of your body. Lie down on the ground taking support of your back and leave your hands and feet loose. Keep a distance of nine inches between the ankles of both the feet.

Let both the arms lie straight on the right and left side of your body comfortably and free from all tension. The hands and fingers should also remain loose. Let the head move freely on its pivot in the vertebral column. Allow your face to move in any direction it chooses. Open your mouth a little bit and let your jaw lie in any position in which it feels convenient. Keep your eyes closed and let your body lie free from all motions.

Hold your breath for a while. After some time release your breath and then breathe inwards. Concentrate your mind on rest so that the nerves may also get complete rest.

This posture removes all kinds of physical and mental fatigue. When the body wilt get rest, its proper development will take place and the height will increase. The fatigue caused by the performance of the earlier movements will totally disappear when you will practise this posture of rest. Hence this posture has been kept in the end of our programme after due consideration.

The practice of this posture is a bit difficult, for we have to control both our mind as well as our body in it. A man or a woman who can take up real rest voluntarily, will find his/ her body always developing (and his/her height will increase as much as possible.) The reason for this is that such a person knows the secret of regaining the energy that has been spent in performing the activities of the day.

The Mid-day

Those men and women, who perform their work by sitting on the chair all the day long and those housewives, who do tailoring or sewing work at home, should perform these movements to make their body long and straighten their waist.

Extension movement while sitting on a chair

Make your legs straight. Also straighten your backbone from waist to neck. Raise your hands straight upwards. Do this for 30 seconds. Repeat it four times.

This will result in the extension of the backbone. The muscles which shrink on account of sitting at one place, get an opportunity of expanding due to this movement.

Straighten your waist

- Take your left hand to your back through your waist and the right hand, over your shoulder to your back and hold the fingers of one hand with the other. Let the palms of both the hands be entangled with each other.
- Pull the palm of the hand below with the palm of the hand above. Thereafter pull the palm of the hand above with the palm of the hand below. Then leave the hands apart.

- Now, take your left hand over your shoulder towards your back and the right hand through the waist to the back and let both the hands meet each other. Now practise the movements 1 and 2 in the reverse order.

The Evening

(1) Come out of your homes for a walk in the evening.

(2) Practise the Movement No.2 meant for women: "Jump and catch the ball." Reduce it in the form of a game.

(3) Lie down on the grass for some time, both on the right as well as on the left sides of your body. The longer you can lie on the grass, the better it would be for improving your height. When your body becomes free from tension, you should practise swinging on a rod.

Some other Useful Exercises

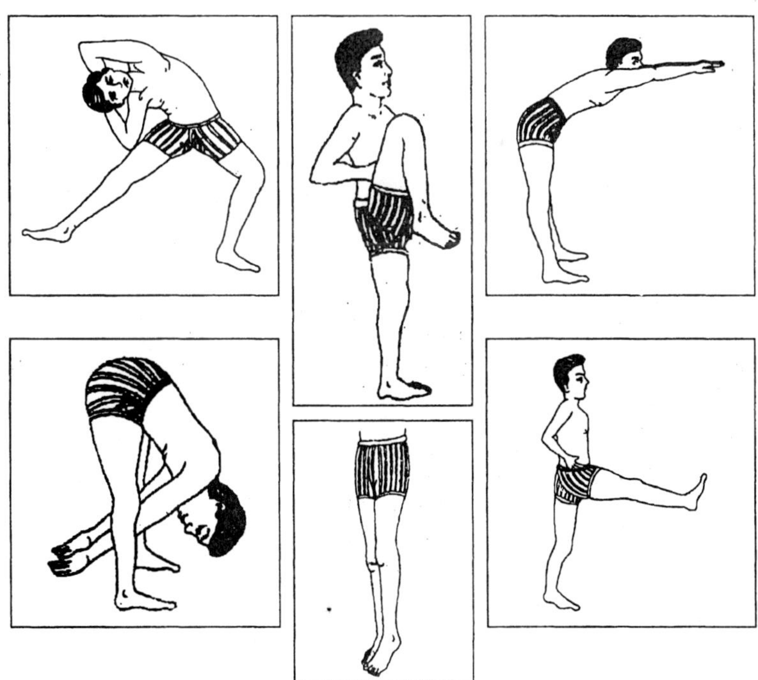

12

Yogasanas to Increase Height

Sarvangasana (Pan Physical Pose)

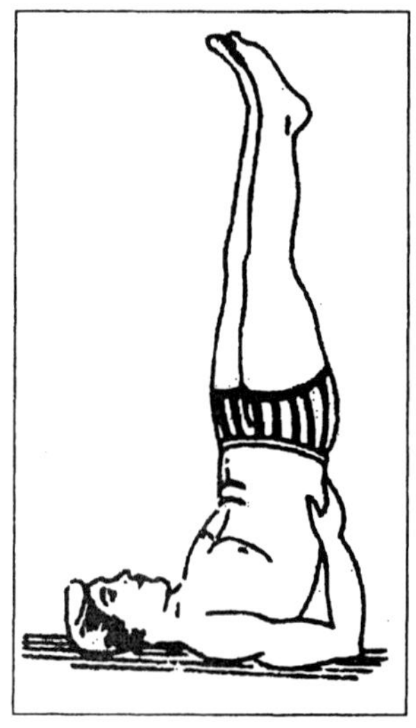

Method—Lie flat on the ground, your spine touching the floor, stretch the body raise the legs slowly and let them stay at right angle to the trunk. After staying for a few seconds slowly raise up the body, without giving any jerk to the spine. Take help from the hands, keeping the fingers outward and thumbs towards the belly. Slowly go on raising the back until the whole trunk is at 90° and the entire weight comes on the shoulders and neck. Take the legs slightly forward and press the chest with your chin. After remaining in the said pose for a few seconds come to the original position.

Benefits—This asana cures constipation, dyspepsia, has a salutary effect on thyroid gland, tones up the nervous system, all limbs of the body, helps to preserve and thicken semen, is useful in intestinal disorders, varicose veins, appendicitis, renders spine flexible, throat disorders are removed, gas is expelled. In addition, it gives glow, vitality and strength to the body, increases sex power, removes menstrual disorders. Persons with hypertension and cordial problems should never take to this asana, except under advice and guidance and supervision of a yoga teacher.

Bhujang or Sarpasana (Cobra/Serpent Pose)

Method—Lie flat on the ground, abdominal portion touching the ground. Straighten both the arms, palms touching the ground. Now bring the palms at level with both sides of abdomen. Slowly lift your neck and torso in such a way that whole body rests on your palms. Now lift your neck upwards gradually and try to look upwards as far and as conveniently you can. Let the toes touch the ground and palms securely resting on the ground. Do not let your elbows bend down. Stay in the position as long you can. When you feel suffocated or when there is a feeling that you can't endure/continue any more, then slowly get back to original position from where you had started. After the asana is over, loosen your limbs and relax.

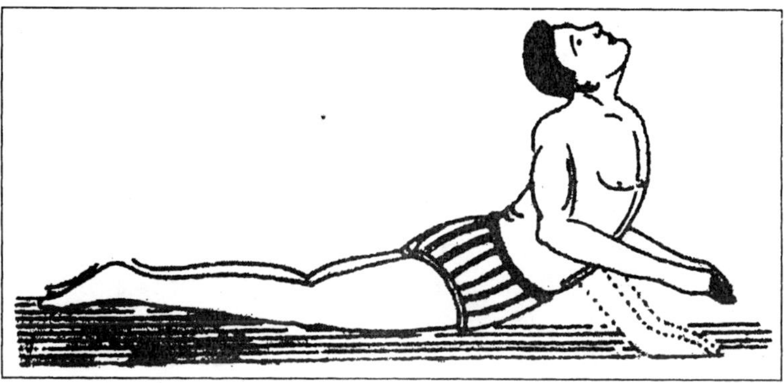

Benefits—Abdominal muscles and back portion are supplied with blood and blood circulation in general, is improved and also fresh and pure blood is supplied to all the organs. It imparts strength, flexibility and tone to spinal column. It removes menstrual disorders and irregularity, helps to improve digestion, chance of night discharge is dispelled, helps to maintain celibacy. It is useful for diabetics, as it activates the pancreas, thereby causing secretion of insulin, render arms, hands and neck painless, flexible and active. Kidneys and intestines also are strengthened.

It removes obesity and sheds extra flesh from the abdominal portion, and spinal curvature and postural abnormalities are also removed.

Chakrasana (A Circle Pose)

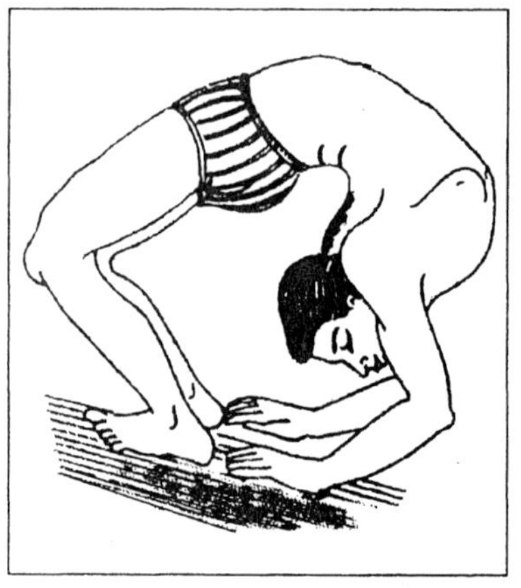

Method—On a hard surface, lie flat on your back. Later, raise the middle portion of your body upwards, fixing and keeping firmly both the feet and hands on the ground thus making a semicircle, ensuring that your head keeps between your hands. Now concentrate your eyes on something that lies in front of you.

Benefits—It enhances, like the sarvanagasana, strength of head, throat, neck, abdomen, legs, hands and, in short, all parts of your body, eliminates pains in joins, removes extra fat from the abdominal area, activates digestive system, renders spinal column elastic and supple, imparts glow and agility to the body, normalises posture and stance, and the body stays erect even during the advanced age. Pregnant ladies should not practice this asana as it can adversely affect their pregnancy process. even leading to miscarriage and bleeding.

Mahavirasana (Named after Lord Mahavir/Hanuman)

Method—Stand erect, bringing forward one foot to a distance of 3 feet from the other. Clench fists of both the hands and raise them. Now, go on jumping alternatively on both the feet, changing the pressure on each feet alternatively. Keep your lips to each other and breath through nose only. When you are tired, take pause until you regain strength to resume the asana. Loosen your limbs and relax.

Benefits—It increases height, sheds extra weight from the waist, body is rendered stronger, chest expands, legs, arms and feet gain strength. It increases sexual power, especially of men, restores normally to menstrual cycle.

Parvatasana

Sit in Padmasana (that is by keeping left foot on the right thigh and right foot on the left thigh). Inhale breath and raise both the hands towards the sky, keeping all the fingers apart and stretching both arms without bending either of them. Stay in the said position as per your capacity and convenience but do not over do. Before you get suffocated, gradually bring down both the arms and place on both the knees and relax, but without binding your back. Keep spinal column erect at 90°. The process can be repeated a number of times. In normal conditions ladies can also perform this asana, but never during pregnancy.

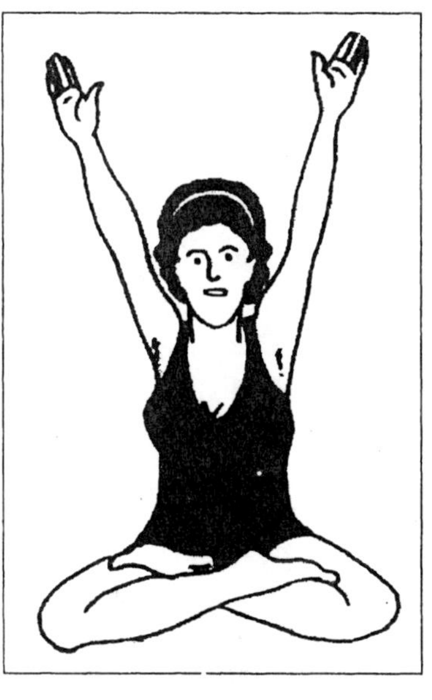

This asana imparts flexibility to the spine, strengthens arms, expands chest, and adds to strength of arms and fingers. Improves flexibility of shoulder blades. It improves upon asthmatic condition and tones up uterus.

Matsyasana

Sit in Padmasana and thereafter lie down on your back. Catch hold of big toe of feet with hands and rise up your back portion in a gradual manner. In this position your backside of head and knees should knees should continue to touch the ground. Retain breath as long you can and stay in the final position and exhale while returning to the previous state.

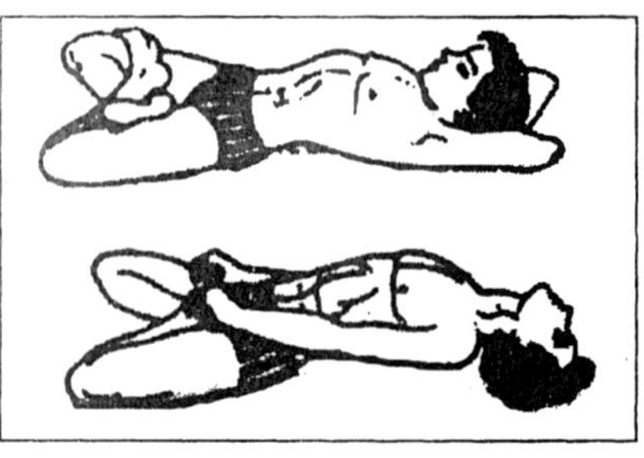

It strengthens chest and lungs, removes extra fat from hips, strengthens legs and hands, dispels asthma, and removes constipation and also column also ensured. In normal health conditions ladies can perform this asana, but not during pregnancy.

Pashchimottanasana

Sit on the floor and spread both legs in front of you and each hold of your big toes with both the hands, but do not let your knees bend. In order to catch the toes you have to bend the back. Initially it may seem slightly difficult to do so, due to rigidity of muscles and limbs; hence do not exert but gradually posture. In 4-5 sitting your body will get attuned to the final posture. Persons with back pain and stiff and muscles, pregnant ladies should not perform this asana unless and until advised by a doctor or yoga expert.

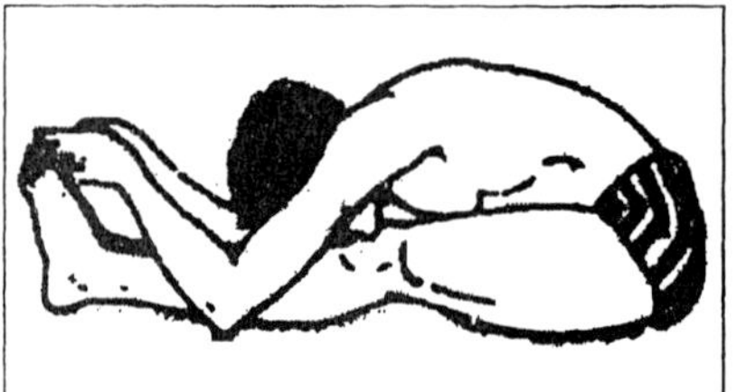

It strengthens legs, arms and renders the spine flexible and supple, improve digestion, removes fat on and around abdomen, constipation fortifies and rejuvenates energy and nervous system, lengthens leg bones, Purifies blood, improves liver, cardiac and respiratory processes, removes fat from hips and sideways.

Note: Those who get adept on this asana, may try to touch their knees with the nose but in the changed position also knees shouldn't be bent.

Ushtrasana

This asana has been named after the camel.

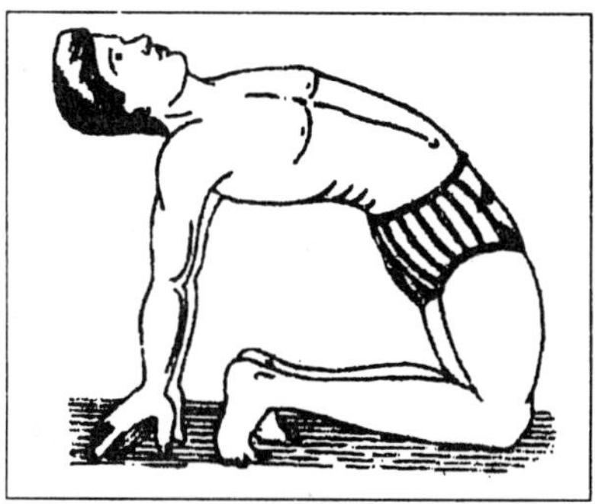

Sit erect and let the weight of entire body fall on both knees and toes of feet. Now catch hold of your heels with the hands, as shown in the figure. While performing this asana, make sure that the back is bent in such a way that neck bends towards feet, back also bends slightly. Look upwards. Stay in the final position as far and as you conveniently can. Retain breath and exhale while getting back to the original (starting) position.

This asana strengthens back, spine, knees, and feet renders spine flexible. After the asana is over, there may be felt ache and stiffness in shoulder blades, knees and feet. To ward off all such effects massage these parts with coconut or mustard oil. Thai asana is capable of increasing height. Pregnant ladies shouldn't perform this asana as it exerts utmost pressure on abdomen and back, but in normal health condition, they may perform this asana, especially when they have backache. Avoid undue pressure and jerk in any case.

Shavasana

Lie down on your back. Keep the whole body loose and in a straights position. Palms can be either on the floor or you can keep them upward. Do not use any pillow under your head.

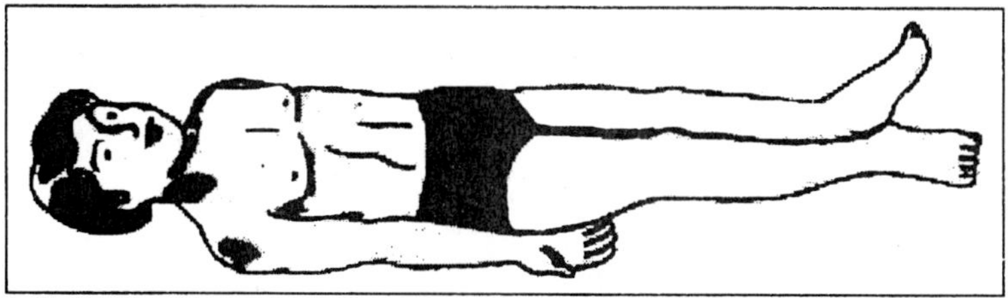

At this point keep breathing in normal way. Keep the eyes closed and let the whole body fall on the floor in an unrestrained way. This position should remain all through the actual practice. This should be done in the last of asanas. This gives us the relaxation.

Yanasana

While performing this asana, body assumes shape and form of a plane flying in the sky; here its nomeclation as such.

Life flats on the floor, while your abdomen touches the ground. Keep both the feet touching each other. First inhale and then raise your head, neck, hands, chest and feet above the ground, keeping all these organs tight and straight-only your abdomen touching the ground. When you feel you cannot retain the inhaled breath. Relax and loosen your limbs. After sometime, it can be repeated 3-4 times or even more, if capacity permits. Even while maintaining normal breath, this asana can also be performed. Pregnant women must never perform this asana.

This asana helps to strengthen bones of arms, hands, shoulders, and legs and also imparts flexibility to the spine. If performed regularly, it can add to inches also. It removes extra fat, improves digestion, removes almost all uterine disorders, and keeps the body supple. This asana is not suitable for pregnant ladies.

Stand erect and keep the feet apart at a distance of 6" to lift. Now gradually bring down the hands and try to touch the ground in front of your toes. While doing so, exert no pressure nor strain unduly. If initially you cannot touch the ground, it is advisable to bend only to the extent possible. As your back and spine become supple, process will look much easier. Do not bend knees, and elbows, keeping your neck straight at 180° while your eyes are affixed looking at the ground or at your hands.

This asana elongates legs and arms, makes spine flexible and supple, improves eyesight, strengthens bones and muscles of legs and hands, and does away with trembling. Persons with backache, hip-joint disease and pregnant ladies must not perform this asana. It also strengths heart, improves cardiac output and efficiency. Improves respiration.

Note—As a general rule any forward bending asana or any physical exercise should never be performed by persons having stiff back, backache and lumbar/spinal spondylysis/curvature. Backward bending asana/exercise may be performed if advised by the concerned experts.

To know more on Asanas, you can read the book of same author, "Pranayama", published by Lotus Press.

■

13

Homoeopathy and Height

Homoeopathy is a science based on symptom—similarity. If you find a good homoeopathic physician in your area, request him to take your case and on totality of your symptoms, he/she can suggest a proper similimum for you.

Baryata carb is a good and leading remedy. Besides, Pitutarin is also a good remedy. There are several other remedies, which can be consulted by your qualified homoeopathic physician.

Ring Fixator Technique

This technique was developed by a Russian Doctor G.A. Ilizarove; during second world war. This technique is used to fix bones of lower extremities and with the same the height can also be improved.

In this process, steal pins of 1.2-1.8 mm. are punctured in leg's bones and are tightened with rings which are worn out side leg. To support these rings, rods too are fixed there. The some can be used to increase length of hands.

This surgery should be performed by a competent orthopaedic surgeon only. Though this is a painful and time consuming technique, but upto four inches height can be increased by this technique.

Besides increasing height, in several bone disorders including multiple fractures, ununiform length of legs/hands, infection of bone etc; this technique is helpful.

■

SLIMMING

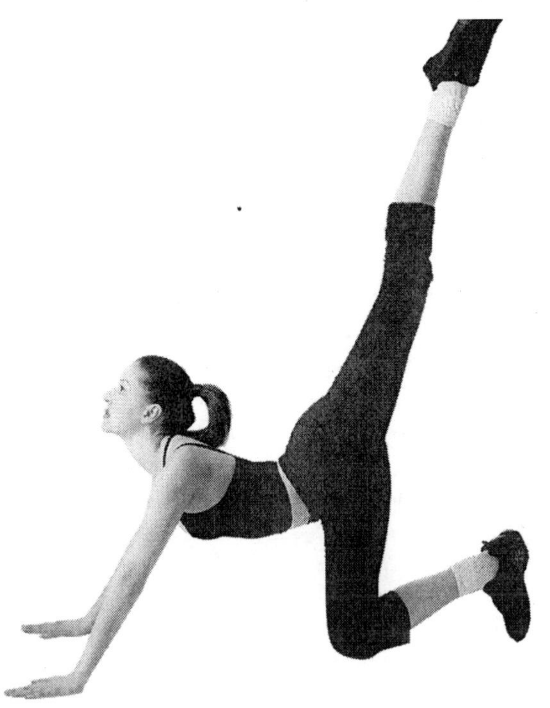

14

Causes and Complications

"It is a condition in which excess fat accumulates in the body, mostly in the subcutaneous tissues. Obesity is usually considered when a person is 20% above the recommended weight for his/her height and build." and how obesity is caused, "The accumulation of fat is caused by the consumption of more food than is required for producing enough energy for daily activities." And also that "obesity is the most common nutritional disorder of recent years."

Obesity is the most common nutritional disorder in affluent societies. Its significance requires constant emphasis because it is associated with increased mortality, predisposes to the development of important diseases and diminishes the efficiency and happiness of those affected and also that "obesity may be defined as a condition in which there is an excessive amount of body fat. This simple definition gives rise to two questions : how can body fat be measured and what is excessive ?"

Conclusions:

1. It (obesity) is a condition of excessive fat accumulation in the body.
2. Fat accumulates in the subcutaneous tissues.
3. A person is obese when he/she weighs 20% above the recommended weight (in relation to his/her height and build).
4. Fat accumulation is caused by excessive intake of food as compared to depleted energy expenses.
5. It (obesity) is a most common nutritional disorder—more particularly of the elite class.

6. It is associated with increased mortality (higher death rate).
7. It is a causative of many killer and non-killer disorders.

Obesity, in itself, is not a disease but it is a most potent factor in causing diseases which are manageable and controllable, provided the obese person adheres to recommended course of dietary regimen, regular and sustainable physical activity, coupled with requisite energy expansion.

Complications triggered by Body of Over Weight

1. Diabetes Mellitus
2. High blood Pressure
3 Arterio-Sclerosis
4. Respiratory problems like breathlessness (dyspnoea) or effort-onset dyspnoea.
5. Early exhaustion and panting even on minimal movement/exertion/effort.
6. Pains and aches in bones, bone-joints, muscles, paving the way for arthritis, osteoarthritis, gout, rheumatism, arthritis deformans, rheumatoid arthritis etc.
7. Acidity, flatulence, colic, constipation or diarrhoea, and other digestion— related disorders.

If we closely look at the information provided above, it is quite easy to conclude that:

(i) Diet

(ii) Exercise or Activity

These are the foremost causatives of overweight but there are still glaring instances when:

- Someone doesn't eat much but is still on the obese side.
- A person may eat more, as a matter of habit, but may not be obese and lead an active life.
- A frail and scarcely built person also may have physical problems, in spite of good food and physical activity.

- Those who eat more are not necessarily overweight and those who eat far less till gain weight.

All the said variable situations do point to one factor, that is eating does not seem to have much relation to overweight but, conversely, it also cannot be denied, on the basis of statistics available, that excessive and frequent intake of food is still considered to be the biggest monster in causing obesity.

Causes of Overweight

This aspect is a ticklish problem, like a crossword puzzle, due to many hypothesis and variant views expressed in this regard. But, there are still some factors over which most of dieticians and doctors agree. Following factors may contribute to excess body fat, leading to overweight and resultant obesity:

1. Overeating
2. Lack of Physical activity
3. Excessive intake of Carbohydrates and Fats
4. Age factor
5. Endocrine glands malfunctioning
6. Heredity

Overeating and Food

Food is meant to generate energy in the body so as to enable each and every body organ to discharge its individual functions. About eating we must not overlook or ignore undernoted points:

(i) Eat only when one is real hungry.

(ii) Eat daily at a fix time.

(iii) Diet should include cereals, pulses, seasonal green and leafy vegetables, fruits, fats (in moderate quantity), milk and milk products etc. In a way daily diet should be a balanced and nutritious diet, consisting of above mentioned food items which should also be rich in minerals and vitamins.

(*iv*) Avoid foods that cause constipation, loose motions, acidity, flatulence, abdominal colic, sour and acidic eructations, belching etc.

(*v*) Avoid foods which are fried and rich in condiments.

(*vi*) Use only unsaturated Vegetable oils like, Soyabean, Sunflower, Palm, Cotton seed oil etc. which reduce cholesterol level.

(*vii*) Avoid using clarified butter, oil, coconut oil, Lard, olive oils and butter which raise cholesterol level, thus causing high blood pressure, cardiac disorders, obesity, joint pains and immobility.

(*viii*) Dietary fibre, obtained from whole grains, vegetables, and fruits should be used in sufficient quantity. Diet, rich in fibre content, is capable of reducing food intake, as it imparts a sense of satiation to the body.

Gluttons must resist the temptation of eating every time. It disturbs the digestive systems and denies rest to digestive organs and other body organs. Labourers, masons, carpenters, persons employed in construction work, mechanics who have to manually operate heavy machinery and equipment, farmers, children in growth-stage, pregnant ladies, lactating mothers. Ladies approaching menopause have to ingest more food than those persons who have to work in an office, shopkeepers, shop employees. If food is not taken in proportion to the expended energy, such a category of persons are liable to get weak but, if persons doing light work also eat heavily, they will be generating more energy which is actually not required.

Operating is also the result of those who sit idle as they have no other activity to perform. Such persons revel in excessive eating as if overeating is the be-all and end-all of their life. When energy is generated through overeating, but no activity is performed to expend the generated energy, it will simply in overweight. For the obese persons overeating is a luxury and a pastime, but for the more hard working persons, sufficient food, to compensate for the energy loss suffered, is a prime necessity.

Calorie Factor

The energy that we derive from diet/food is measured as 'Calorie' which, in fact, is an energy measuring unit and the calories burnt (during the course of physical exercise and exertion). Number of calories burnt/expended, amount of labour put in to a discharge one's work in relation to age, sex, climate. A child, during the growth stage and also during playing games, an old person leading a sedentary life style, a person working in an office, a manual labourer, a stone-cutter, tree-feller, a pregnant woman, during and after pregnancy, a hospitalised patient will require different percentage of calories. Simple rule is: the more energy one spends, the higher calories he would require. When we talk of calorie, total calories required by a person during duration of 24 hours will be reckoned by total calories, obtained from various sources of nutrition. Two persons of the same height, age and workload, would require, different amount of calories because metabolism of each person differs. Every one is a law unto himself, when above criteria are taken into consideration. Two main groups, viz. vegetarians and non-vegetarians, have to work out food items which, when combined, give total calories required by a person. There is another class which adheres to both the said types of food categories.

As already indicated, a balanced diet must be a unified entity, consisting of cereals, green vegetables, fibre, fruits, milk and its various products, meats etc. so that the dietary intake presents a homogenous combination of essential carbohydrates, proteins, fats, minerals, vitamins etc. It is a myth that costly foods give better nutritious values than the cheaper ones but, luckily, the facts is the other way round. So, when working out on your food and diet, you should be more conscious of the nutritional factor than the cost factor. Main purpose is and should be to meet calorie requirement of the body than the money spent therefore.

Dietary Fibre

Fibre is the material which makes the cell walls in the plants and is the indigestible portion thereof. It is neither absorbed by the body nor can it be broken down by the enzymes. In earlier days, it was considered to be a useless matter and was not accorded and therapeutic usage and utility. But, the actual position is that if fibre is discarded and eliminated from our diet, water cannot hold on to the body, thus causing dryness of faeces which results in constipation. It also helps in free movement of intestines and almost rules out inflammation and dryness of intestines, alongwith accumulation of toxi subsistence therein.

Fibre is found in two major kinds: Soluble and insoluble. Certain vegetables and grain cereals have more insoluble fibre. Barley, oats, legumes and fruits contain more soluble fibre. The former (Insoluble fibre) aids in removing costiveness and improves digestion, whereas the latter (soluble fibre) helps to lower the serum cholesterol but raises proportion of the good cholesterol, HDL (High Density Lipoprotiens).

In support of our opinion we would like to add Dr. Bukitt's expert opinion. "Diets, high in fibre and low in fat, yield soft, moist and plentiful stools, eliminate the need for straining, and are of great help in preventing and treating not only constipation, but (also) haemorrhoids and varicose veins." High fibre diets are required to be chewed for a longer time and, more the time is spent in chewing, the less amount of food intake would ensue. It will also give satisfaction and sweetish taste, by constant mixing of saliva, resulting in quick and proper digestion. Since fibres lower insulin levels and thus, lowered insulin secretion will not stimulate appetite. The general rule, in this regard, is that the more the insulin, the more the appetite, and more the appetite, the more intake of food—the last one being the reason for obesity, diabetes and other disorders. So, one can easily infer and deduce that high fibre foods would reduce dietary intake. High soluble fibre foods stay for longer time in the stomach and, thus, there is a feeling of satiated fullness. Above reasons would suffice to justify an intake of high fibre foods in greater quantity so as to shed weight and stay trim.

"Fibre discourages us from eating more than we (actually) need. Fibre is unique in that it satiates but does not supply calories." If you take juice of two apples and eat two apples, you will feel that, after taking juice, you are again ready to eat, but not so after eating apples and the biggest surprise is that difference is only of 3 gms of fibre per 100 gms of juice/raw apples.

Fibre is a bulking agent. It helps information of stool and renders it bulkier. For smooth passage of stools, it is essential that it should be soft, compact, bulky and smooth so that it passes through the rectum without pain, exertion or strain.

Highly fat-rich foods/diets should be replaced by high fibre diets, especially by heart and cancer patients (in case they are not bed-ridden or inactive). Dr. Burkitt opines thus: "A high fibre diet tends to lower the blood pressure of hypertensive patients", "Research has shown that pectin, the fibre found in the skin of fruits, vegetables and sunflower seeds, will lower blood cholesterol levels." (Quoted respectively from British Med. Journal and American Journal of Clinical Nutrition).

Lack of Physical Activity

Labourers and others, performing vigorous activity need not undertake any extra exercise, as the jobs done by them suffice to expend the calories. The main problem lies with easy chaired persons, office workers, shop girls/boys who have to stand for long hours, elite people, sedentary and inactive housewives, children who do not play any game or exercise.

Advantages of Physical Activity

1. Helps to keep digestive system in functional condition.
2. Tones up circulation of blood.
3. Maintains flexibility of body.
4. Improves cardiac rhythm and output.
5. Helps in normal respiration.
6. Energies blood vessels and doesn't allow cholesterol deposit therein.
7. Improves skin condition, improves complexion, opens up pores of the skin and lets out toxins through sweating.
8. Removes constipation and improves peristaltic action of intestines, rectum and anus.
9. Doesn't allow muscles and joints to become rigid.
10. Dispels pains and aches in body organs, by feeding them with fresh body supply.
11. Tones up nervous system.
12. Doesn't allow extra fat to accumulate.

Ways to Maintain Physical Activity

- Daily morning walk and stroll after taking dinner.
- Attending to calls of nature, taking bath, maintaining a high standard of personal hygiene.
- Performing Pranayamaa and Yogasanas.
- Aerobic exercise or Push-up exercises.
- Maintaining regularity in daily chores and doing job-related work.
- Not sticking to one posture for longer period.
- Cycling, running, gymnastic exercises.
- Playing games, like badminton, tennis, football, hockey, cricket, kho-kho, kabaddi, swimming, table tennis, jumping, skipping etc.

Remember, playing cards, chess, carrom board, video games, watching TV/Movies, reading newspapers, gossiping, sitting idle for hours together, doing desk-work etc. do not form part of physical activity. In fact these help to add weight to body, hence these are impediments to healthy living and are not only injurious to health but an open invitation to host of diseases which could have been averted, if a person starts doing anyone of the exercise patterns described above.

Hazards of Inactivity

(i) Disturbed digestion.

(ii) Cardiac or Pulmonary dyspnoea.

(iii) Blood Pressure, headache, aching in eyes, and tiredness thereof.

(iv) Rough skin with foul-smelling perspiration or even total/partial absence of perspiration.

(v) Pain and stiffness in neck, shoulders, arms, hands, upper and lower back, hip-joint, knees, legs and feet.

(vi) Even minimal efforts brings on fatigue, soreness, lethargy and there is total dis-inclination even to moderate activity.

(vii) General weakness, rundown condition, apathy, indifference, agitated behaviour, easy proneness to infection.

(viii) Low physical resistance and body's defence mechanism is thrown to shambles.

(ix) Nerves, muscles and bones cry for nutritional supplementation.

Who should Perform Exercises

Any healthy person of any age should not hesitate to perform anyone of the exercise related activities which must commensurate with amount of food intake and nature of job. Sports persons and athletes have been seen to be quite regular in taking exercise daily. Housewives who perform all or most of the domestic chores need not take to any extra physical activity since dusting, cleaning of floor, washing clothes, making purchases from the market are sufficient activities for them to keep fit and healthy.

Children and young persons should play outdoor games and sports to keep fit and expend the energy and also that their diet also must be such as to meet requirements at the growth stage. They should resist from playing indoor games (except table tennis, if played in a room or courtyard). Moreover they must develop the habit of doing their own work themselves, instead of depending on their family members or servants.

For old and aged persons early morning walk and simple stroll after dinner will suffice to meet their demands on physical activity, provided they do not suffer from any incapacitating disorder. If they are unable to resort to walking, they should simply perform Pranayamaa and other breathing exercises and also light physical exercises which do not interfere with their physical status/disability. But they must avoid any activity where jerks or falls are feared or anticipated. Even bathing is a good exercise for them, but heart patients must consult their doctors before taking to any activity.

You may or may not derive desired results by doing any physical activity or advantages may be noticed quite late, if done properly but, an exercise done wrongly is bound to harm the body. Adventurous games like trekking, hill climbing, swimming, some aerobic exercises should be done under guidance of the concerned coach.

Persons Who should Avoid Physical Activity

Persons who suffer from acute attack of asthma, severe and excruciating headache, backache, stiff and totally immobile joints, in febrile conditions, cancer of any aetiology, after any operation, during the course of travelling, mental agitation, pregnant ladies, debilitated and incapacitated old persons, weak and undernourished children/young persons, stomach ulcers, cirrhosis and cancer of liver, heavy drunkards, chain smokers, drug addicts, traumatic cases should not perform any physical activity or exercise without advice of the attending doctor. If they take to any physical activity of their own, they are simply inviting a calamity for themselves and a problem for other house inmates.

Similarly, no exercise should be performed immediately after return from daily work, in extreme cold, heat and moist weather and when it is raining. Patients to asthma and other respiratory disorders are warned not to venture in performing any physical exercise/vigorous activity when there is an acute attack. Further, when the body is drenched with preparations, when breathlessness sets in, when visibility is poor, weather conditions are not congenial, when stomach is full, or after prolonged fasting. These unfavourable conditions apply to all age groups and both the sexes.

Excessive Intake of Fats

Fat is an essential part of our diet and it is height of imprudent discretion to totally eliminate fats from daily diet. For a normal diet daily consumption of 25 gms is a usual standard requirement. Only saturated fats cause havoc in the form of raised serum cholesterol level which results in raised blood pressure, arteriosclerosis, coronary heart disease, excessive fat accumulation in the body which is the prime factor in obesity and overweight.

Carbohydrates are obtained from sugar, rice, wheat, jaggery, fruits and some vegetables and energy to body is provided by them. It is a fact that heat generated by fats is almost double the amount of energy generated by carbohydrates. Fats are also essential for mobility of joints. But, in order to digest the fats, rigorous and hard activity is required. Excessive ingestion of fats and carbohydrates is responsible for adiposity (obesity).

Fats discharge following functions viz.:

1. To provide protection to body organs.
2. To store energy in the body.
3. To promote growth of body organs by providing necessary fats, and
4. To retain the generated head within the body.

Excessive fat consumption finds its way through stools as it is not absorbed within the body. Fat and overweight persons have immense capacity to eat and also digest, and this is the reason as to why fat accumulates in their bodies. It is a fashion in elite and well to do families to eat fat-rich friend foods which are overloaded with carbohydrates also.

There are 3 types of fats viz:

(i) Saturated Fats—These are (saturated) fatty acids that raise serum cholesterol level.

(ii) Polyunsaturated Fats—These fats do not raise serum cholesterol levels.

(iii) Monosaturated Fats—These fats bring down serum cholesterol level and are also known to raise HDL.

Following comparative table will clearly show presence of above mentioned types of fats.

Percentage of Various types of Fat found in Oils

S. No.	Fats oils	Saturated Fatty Acids	Mono unsaturated Fatty Acids	Poly unsaturated Fatty Acids
1.	Butter oil	65	37	4
2.	Coconut oil	91	6	3
3.	Corn oil	13	26	61
4.	Cotton seed oil	28	19	53
5.	Lard	43	45	12
6.	Olive oil	53	37	10
7.	Peanut oil	18	49	33
8.	Sunflower oil	11	22	67
9.	Soyabean oil	16	24	60
10.	Sesame oil	16	41	43
11.	Mustard Oil	-	-	25
12.	Rice Bran	-	-	35
13.	Vanasapati	-	-	6

Note: Mark—denotes Fat Contents not known.

30% of total calorie requirement should be met through unsaturated fatty acids and not from saturated ones. It is necessary that total intake of unsaturated fats should be equally spread over and divided within a period of 24 hours so that there is a regular supply of such fats to all the body organs and production of energy is also uniform. In any case a normal person may consume 25-30 gms of fats daily in divided ones. The said quantity may be raised in the case of persons doing strenuous manual work, irrespective of sex and age.

Carbohydrates

Optimum energy is generated by carbohydrates in the body. Crystal sugar, jaggery, barley, gram, corn/maize, rice, sugars obtained from vegetables (like beets, sweet potato etc), fruits like grapes, mangoes, cherry, apricot, dates, raisins, coconut (fresh), currants, apples, oranges, sweet lime etc. Carbohydrates obtained from fruits metabolise quickly as compared to the ones generated by grain cereals. In diabetes carbohydrates, in excessive quantity, are prohibited but must not be totally eliminated from daily diet. Milk, cheese, yeast, honey have also carbohydrates whereas cow's/goat's milk, Yogurt have low calorie carbohydrates. In obesity, role of carbohydrates cannot be denied.

If a person consumes too much of carbohydrates and fat containing food, his weight is bound to increase. If an ailing and bed-ridden patient resorts to too much intake of carbohydrates, but is not in a position to take to physical activity, he is bound to gain weight and may even become a diabetic or, at least, get prone to the risk of diabetes.

Malfunctioning of Endocrine Glands

An endocrine influence on body fat is seen both in normal physiological situations and in pathological states. The normal content of young adult woman is twice that of youngman, and pregnancy is characterised by an increase in body weight. Obesity in woman commonly begins at puberty, during pregnancy or at the menopause. Obesity frequently, but not invariably, accompanies hypothyroidism, hypogonadism, hypopituitarism and cushing's syndrome. However, the overwhelming majority of obese patients show no clinical evidence of an endocrine disorder. Plasma insulin and cortisol are commonly raised and growth hormone reduced in obese subjects, but these changes probably result from, rather than cause, the obesity, since they disappear when weight is lost.

Hypothyroidism is not a decided factor in causing obesity, though, in some obese patients it is also the cause. Deficiency of this hormone can be effectively met with administration of tablets of thyroxine (available in 25, 50, 100 mg tablets) but strictly under medical advice and supervision.

Age Factor

Obesity is generally prevalent in middle age, but it could occur at any stage of life. Weight gain at pregnancy, after delivery, at the time of or after menopause, is quite common. But if a child or adolescent becomes obese at these stages, he will most likely remain an obese in adult life also. After delivery most ladies, irrespective of age, have heavier buttocks, thick thighs, pendulous abdomen and large-sized breast, and all these changes help them towards obesity but, during course of time, most of them regain their former weight, if they continue with recommended exercises. Persons suffering from gout and other disabilities put on extra weight due to lack or absence of physical activity - here age is no bar. If a crippling disability afflicts a person, he can gain weight at any stage of life.

Heredity

It is not necessary that obese parents will necessarily have obese children. Even twin babies do not have an identical weight. Similarly, slim and trim parents also have obese children and vice versa. But genetic and environmental factors do play an important role, as effects of environment, in certain regions of our country, daily use of carbohydrates and fats is customary and inmates of such areas are seen to be generally obese. There is no denying fact that food habits play a significant role in pushing up weight. During the last 25 years, there has been a progressive increase in the percentage of obese and overweight people. Children of obese parents have high risk factor in inheriting obesity from their parents but, even then, exceptions are still many.

■

15

Sundry Causes of Obesity

Socio-Economic Factors

Obesity is more common in lower socioeconomic groups of affluent countries, but in developing countries obesity is more common in the prosperous elite class. occupations of cooks and barmen are more prone to obesity while front desk receptionists, fashion designers, models, air hostesses, airline pilots, society girls have to keep slim and trim figures. Similarly, film actors and actress, extras, society girls, call girls, prostitutes have also to keep themselves slim to ensure themselves a longer stay in their respective professions.

In some societies fat women and men earn a place of status and are respected but, in others, fat people are neither respected nor considered attractive.

Drugs

Use of oral contraceptives, steroids, insulin and phenothiazines is generally followed by weight gain due to stimulation of appetite. When indoor patients are kept on medication for longer period, their weight normally does not increase but, after their return to homes, they start to take prescribed medicines—it is as if a convict has been released from a jail and, in a spirit of vengeance, he throws all the earlier imposed restrictions to winds and feels free to eat any type of food.

Alcohol

Alcohol as such, may not be a precipitating factor in causing rise in body-weight but drunkards usually follow drinks with meat/fish, fried and heavily spiced vegetables, rice or bread, extra fats in the form of butter, clarified butter, dry fruits. Heavy meals is not uncommon in drunkards as, when in a drunken state, they cannot distinguish between good or bad food, which food is harmful and what quantity is actually needed. Operating is a consequence of drinking, followed by rise in body weight, acidity, vomiting, sour and acidic eructations, flatulence, abdominal colic etc.

Fasting

Fasting is a cleansing process which helps to divest the body from harmful toxins and also affords well deserved rest and holiday from diet consumption, even though for a specific period only. It is held that no food should be taken during fasting but some people do take ice-creams, cold drinks, sweetmeats, sweets, chocolates, so that 'they don't feel weak'. Ladies, though not all, utilise fasting as an effective means to satiate their hunger for abundant rich diet, and also do not hesitate to ingest even the prohibited foods. All these habits lead one to obesity.

Tendency to Obesity

In certain families obesity can be commonly seen and the reasons for putting on extra weight are too many to count. Despite best efforts, there is no shedding of weight. Here genetic factor could be the possible factor in adding to body weight. It is not that excessive food intake is generally the contributory cause, apart from sedentary life style. Obese parents can, at least, educate, motivate and guide their siblings about hazards of overweight. It would be still better, if parents and elderly people invite the young ones to join them in weight reducing exercises.

■

16

Facts About Cholesterol

Cholesterol is a fatty substance found in the human body and in foods that come from animals. It has many positive functions within the body and is required for us to be healthy. However, too much cholesterol in the blood can be unhealthy. Cholesterol constitutes a major component of the plaque build-up that occurs in the arteries. This plaque narrows the arteries and can eventually lead to coronary artery disease. A diet high in fat, especially saturated fat, significantly contributes to unhealthy levels of cholesterol in the body.

Cholesterol Tests

Your doctor can use a blood test to measure your total blood cholesterol, your high-density lipoprotein (HDL) and low-density lipoprotein (LDL) cholesterol levels, and also your triglycerides.

- **Total blood cholesterol:** A total blood cholesterol level less than 200 mg/dL is desirable. This level of total cholesterol is associated with the least risk of heart disease.
- **HDL ("good") cholesterol:** HDL cholesterol is known as "good" cholesterol because a high level seems to protect us against heart attacks by carrying cholesterol away from your arteries. On the average, men should have HDL cholesterol levels ranging from 40 to 50 mg/dL, and women should have levels ranging from 50 to 60 mg/dL. A HDL cholesterol level less than 40 mg/dL is considered low.
- **LDL ("bad") cholesterol:** LDL cholesterol can slowly build up on the walls of the arteries that feed the heart and brain. LDL cholesterol is known as "bad" choles-

terol because a high level indicates an increased risk of heart disease. A LDL cholesterol level less than 130 mg/dL is desirable.

- **Triglycerides:** High triglyceride levels often appear with higher levels of total cholesterol and LDL cholesterol, and low levels of HDL cholesterol. A normal triglyceride level is considered to be less than 150 mg/dL.

Controlling Cholesterol Levels

You can lower your blood cholesterol level by losing weight (if needed), exercising and eating healthful foods.

Diets high in fat, particularly saturated fat, and cholesterol raise blood cholesterol levels. A few simple modifications in your diet can help you control your cholesterol level. By following these simple guidelines, you will find that a diet low in fat and cholesterol can be easy and delicious:

- Eat more fish, skinless poultry and lean cuts of meat (trim all visible fat).
- Eat more fruits, vegetables and grains.
- Cook with unsaturated vegetable oils instead of butter.
- Choose skim or 1% milk, and low fat dairy products.
- Limit consumption of egg yolks to three or four per week, or use egg whites and egg substitutes in place of whole eggs.

■

17

Dieting Without Exercises

One may ask the question that if fat can be got rid of by dieting (reducing intake of calories) then why should one exercise.

The answer to this query is that nearly all the medical experts agree that obesity or fatness is caused not merely by one factor. That is, that we take more calories than we bum out. The muscles and tissues that we generally not use also convert themselves into fat.

If a person does dieting without proper exercises, he would merely be a 'lean weak person' instead of 'fat weak person.' This does not indicate any improvement in health. As a matter of fact, such a person feels more tension and pressure on his body and hence becomes peevish. The resistance power of his body against diseases also dimin ishes. He falls an easy prey to diseases. Not only that, he tires very quickly. Dieting without proper exercises may result in many complications and may prove harmful. If you reduce the intake of food without exercising the body, the bodily energy gets less and the flexibility of muscles is also diminished. It has been proved by experiments that if you do dieting accompanied by proper exercises, then the fat in .your body is evenly distributed to every part of it The body becomes well-proportioned and attractive. Every muscle of the body becomes active and energetic. Due to better circulation of blood during exercises, your face becomes youthful. Due to quick and rapid breathing, the toxic elements in the body get burnt out and the body becomes free of all diseases. You inhale 417 grains of oxygen per hour when you are relaxing. On the other hand, the intake of oxygen during exercises is increased to 1830 grains per hour.

The toxic elements of the body also come out of the body in the shape of perspiration during exercise.

The movement of all parts of body during exercise increases the appetite and aids digestion. Every thing that you eat is easily digested and is retained by the body. The metabolism of the body improves. Exercise helps the body to assimilate useful elements from the food which are then not thrown out in the form of toxic matters. The extra fat on many parts of the body is burnt. If you exercise, you aid every cell of the body in getting its nutrition. The fat melt.., during the exercises and is then evenly distributed amongst different.parts of the body. Hence, you can only aim to have a well-proportioned and attractive figure, if you do exercises along with dieting to get rid of your extra weight and fat. The movement of the body aids in destroying the unwanted and harmful ingredients of the food and thus nullifies their evil effects.

Exercise without Dieting

If you do regular exercises without any dieting, it shall cause no evil effect. On the other hand, it shall remove the looseness of the body and induce tightness. Gradually,the fat will be dissolved and every part of the body will become well-shaped. But, this shall take a long time. You will feel the effect after years of regular exercises. Your aim is to have a shapely, well-proportioned and attractive figure by reducing your weight and obesity in a few months. You can get ridof your ugly fat only if you do regular exercises accompanied by dieting.

■

18

Exercises for Different Body Parts

For moulding and strengthening hips, thighs, abdomen, waist, arms and breasts

Do the exercises given on the next few pages, regularly for fifteen minutes daily. You will find your unwanted fat disappearing and your weight will go down by 11 to 16 kilograms in just one-and-a-half month. You will start seeing the results of this routine after a week. If these exercises are performed with music playing in the room, you will enjoy them more. When you have mastered these exercises say in, two weeks, you can increase the duration to half an hour. But, this should be done gradually. When you have got rid of the extra ungainly fat and weight, continue doing these exercises to retain a well-proportioned and balanced body. Make these exercises a daily habit.

Exercises for Waist

- Stand near a wall with your left shoulder pointing towards the wall. The left hand should be stretched at the height of your shoulder. Rest the left hand on the wall. Move away your waist from the wall as far as you can. Your right arm should be extended above your head with your palms pointing towards the ceiling. Move your body twice away from the wall. Rest your right hand on your

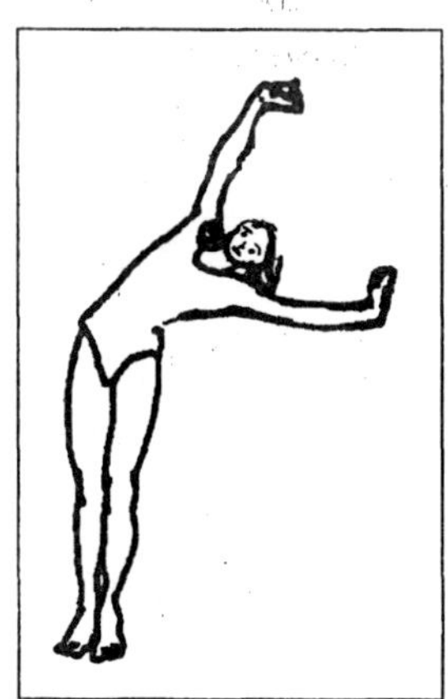

waist. Press your body towards the wall twice and repeat this exercise fifteen times.

- *Stand erect.* Hold a wooden rod with both the hands at your back, as given in the illustration. The legs should be apart from each other. Now move your body to left in circular motion. Bring back the body to the straight position and then move it to the right. Then, resume the straight position. Repeat this exercise fifteen times.

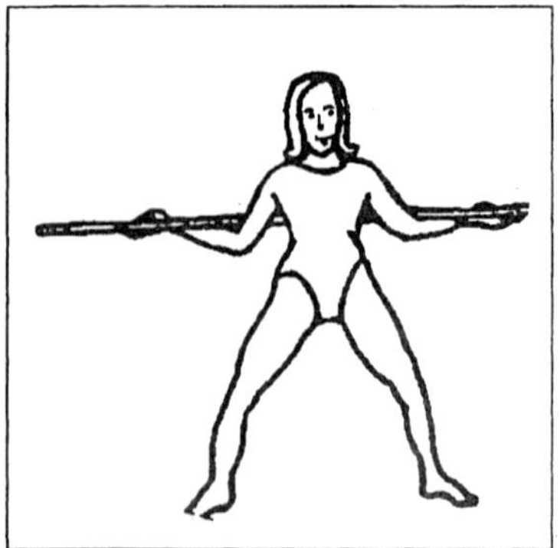

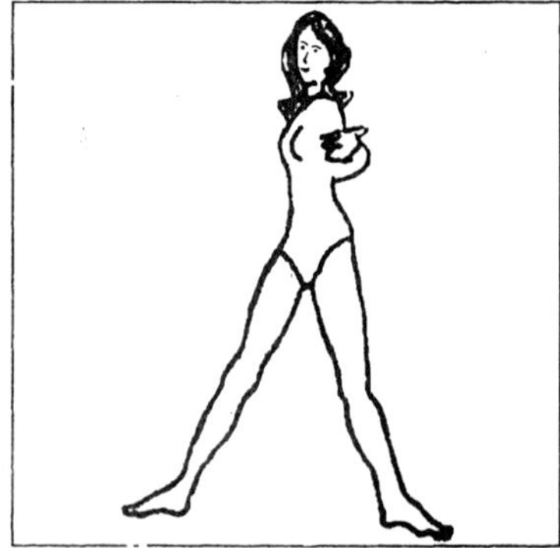

- Hold the wooden rod in both your hands at your back. Keep the legs far apart. Tighten the muscles of hips and buttocks. Draw the abdomen inside trying to bring it as close to the back as possible. Now, turn the body to the left and then right. Do this for fifteen times.

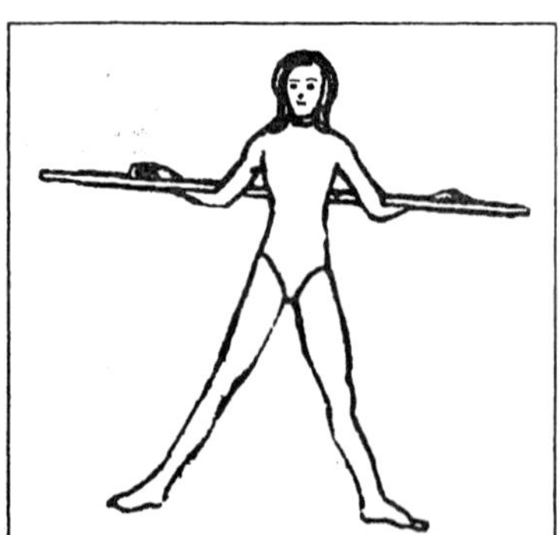

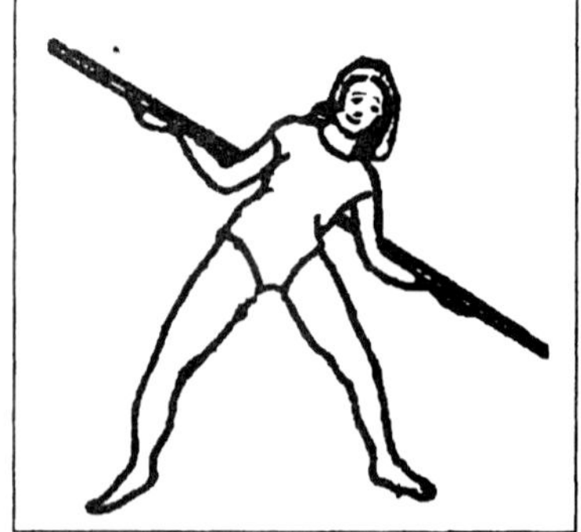

(a) *(i)* *Stand erect.* keep the legs apart. Stretch the right arm to the right and left arm to the left.

(ii) Bend the body from the waist. Extend both the arms upwards.

(iii) Jump up and stand erect. Repeat this exercise four time.

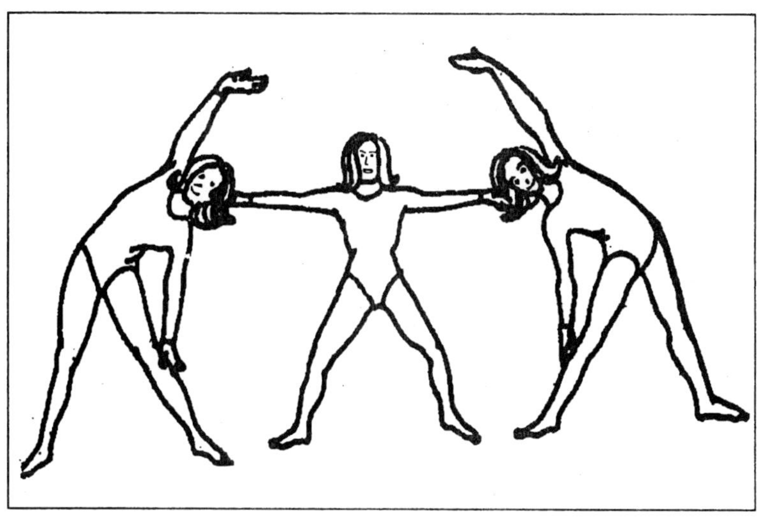

(b) *(i)* Bend towards left. Extend the left arm downwards. The right arm is to be extended upwards.

(ii) Resume the first position. Do this exercise three times.

(iii) Now bend towards the right with right arm stretched, downwards. The left arms should be stretched upwards as in the illustration. Repeat it three times.

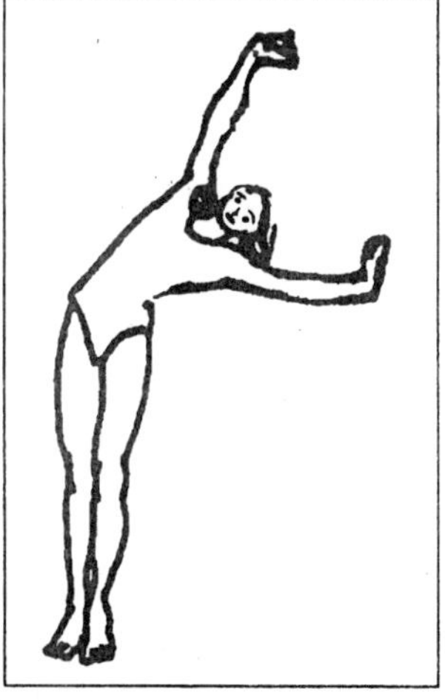

Abdominal Exercises

1. Lie on your back. keep both the hands under the hips. Stretch both the legs straight on the ground. Lift both the legs slowly towards the ceiling. The feet should be stretched inwards while the heels are pointing out.

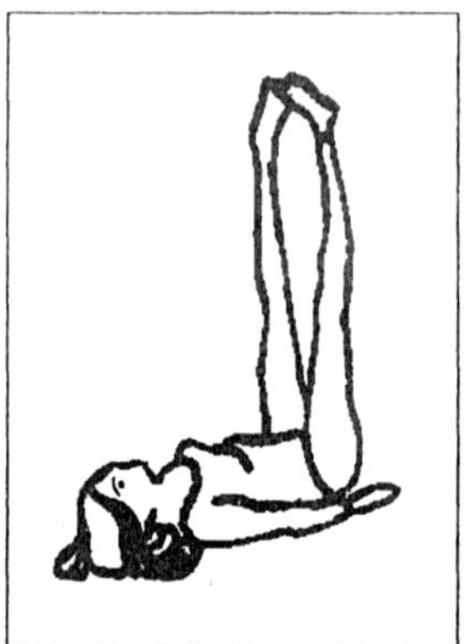

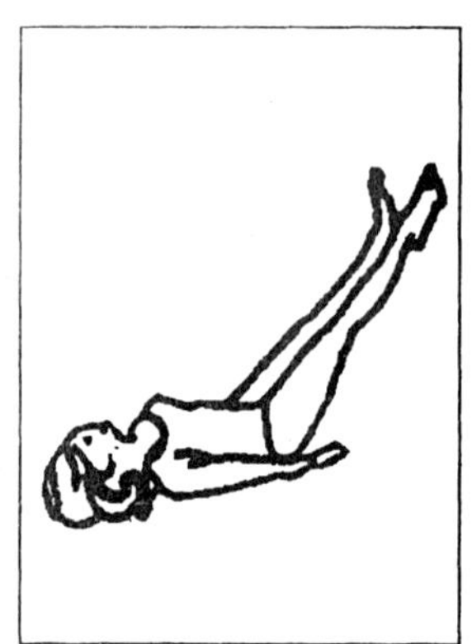

Bring down the legs. Keep them at an angle of 45 degrees. Stretch the feet outwards. Press the heels inwards. Bring down the legs to the ground. Repeat it fifteen times.

2. Lie on your back. Keep the hands under the hips. Lift the head and legs about six inches above the ground. Remain in this position for ten seconds. Head and legs should remain above the ground. Bend the knees and bring them close to your chest. Rest for five seconds and then repeat this exercise thrice.

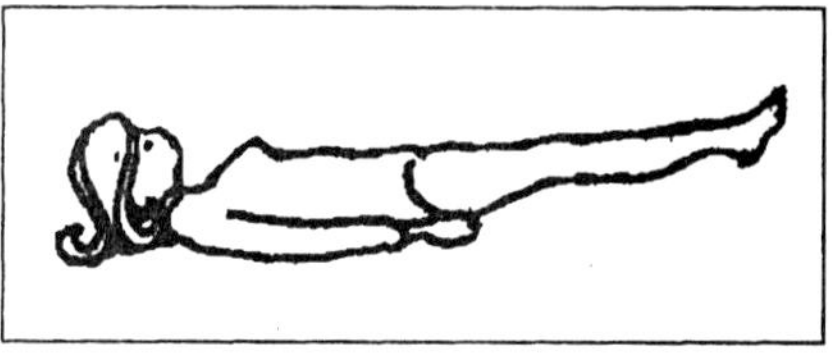

3. Rest your elbows on the ground. The upper part of your body should be in a raised position. Lift both the legs a few inches above the ground. Try to pull the abdomen inwards.

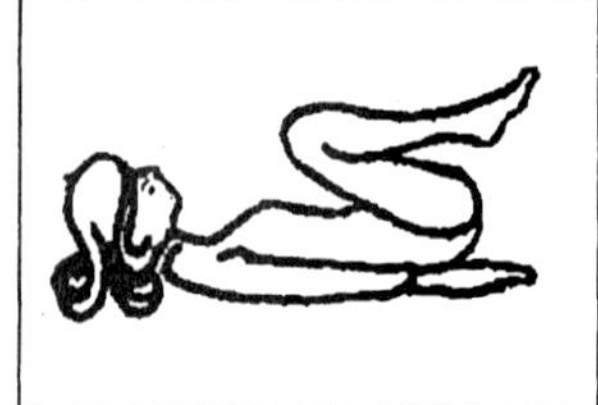

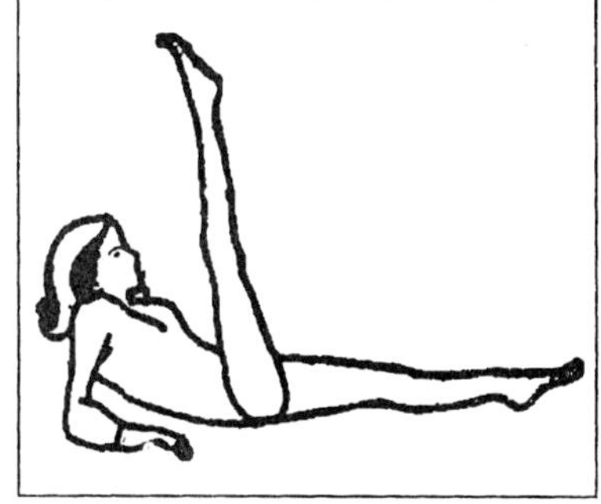

(*a*) Lift the left leg towards the ceiling (upwards). The right leg should remain in a slightly raised position. It should not touch the ground.

(*b*) Now, raise the right leg towards the ceiling and see to it that the left leg remains extended in the front and does not touch the ground. Repeat this exercise with each leg at least fifteen times.

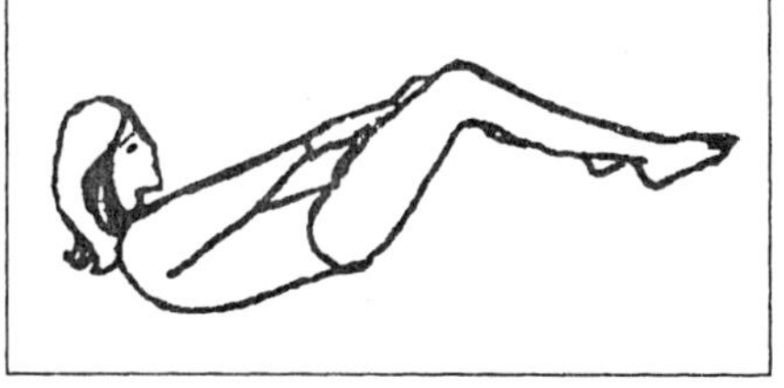

4. (*a*) Sit on the ground and extend the legs. The knees should be in a half-bent position. Now try to lie down very slowly. The backbone of the spinal column should rest on the ground. The head and shoulders should be in a raised position. Extend your arms in front of yourself.

(*b*) Now jump forward. The upper part of your body should be above the ground while the waist touches the ground. Repeat it ten times.

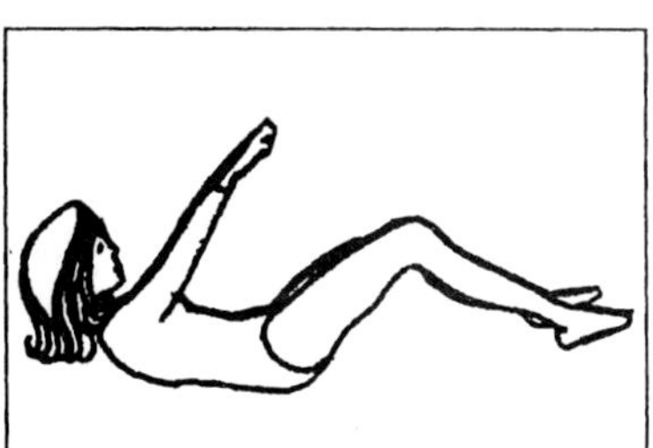

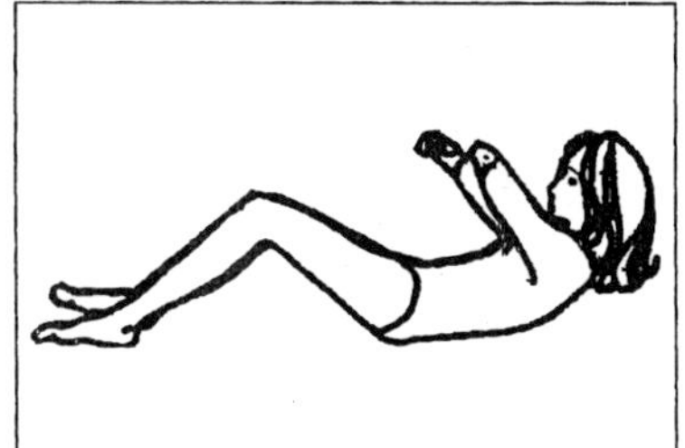

5. Lie on your back. The knees should be apart from each other in half bent position. The head and shoulders should be in a raised position. Extend the right arm towards left and the left arm towards right above your chest. Then, extend both the arms fully infront of you. The right arm should be on the right side while the left arm should be towards the left. Repeat it ten times. While extendeing the arms, raise the upper part of your body from the ground. Take care that the lower part of your hips remain in touch with the ground.

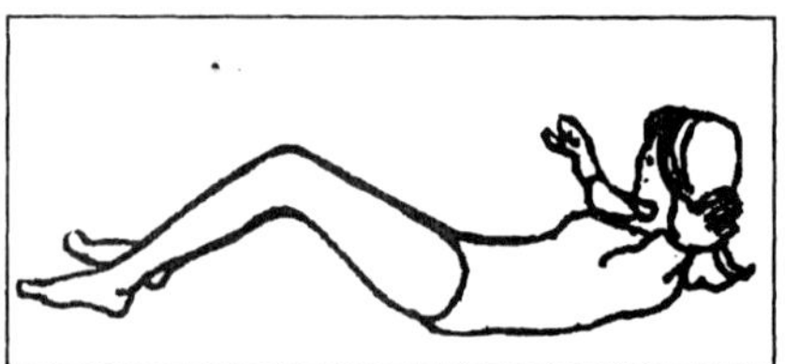

6. Lie on your back. Extend both the legs upwards an4 rest them on a wall. Extend both the arms towards your head. Take forward your arms towards the legs. Jump forward five times. Take some rest and then again jump five times. Rest and then repeat it three times.

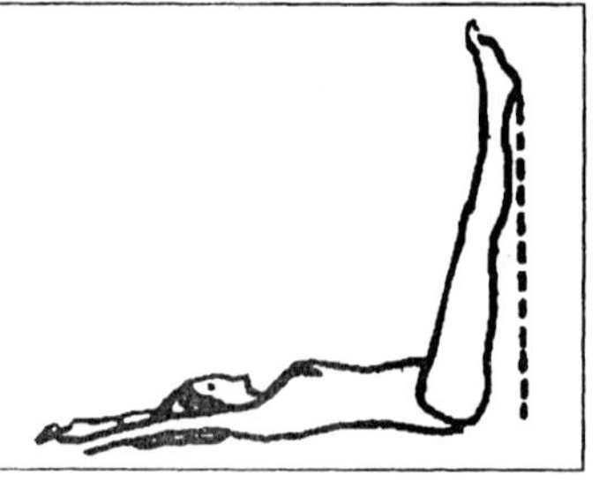

Remember: The legs should be absolutely straight.

7. *(a)* Sit down. Extend your legs straight in front. The back should be straight. The legs should be a little apart. Hold a wooden stick with both your hands. The arms should be at a distance of three feet from each other. Bring your arms from your back to over your

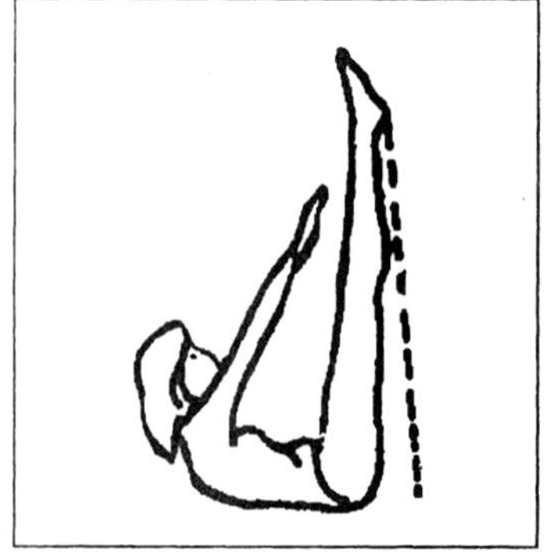

head, holding the wooden stick in your hands. Try to take the wooden stick as high as possible over the head. Now bring the wooden stick in front of you. At the same time raise your left leg towards the wooden stick.

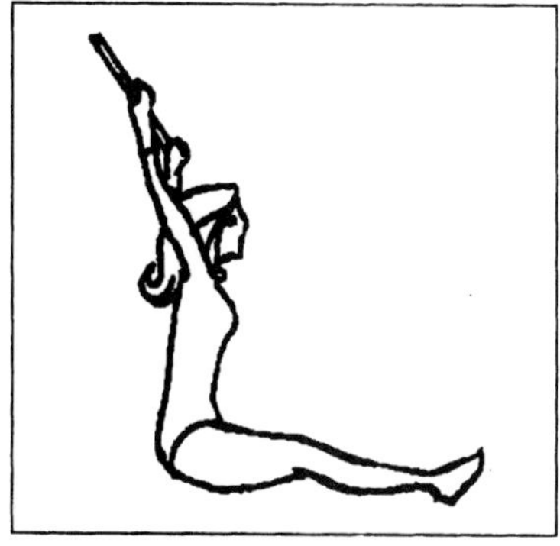

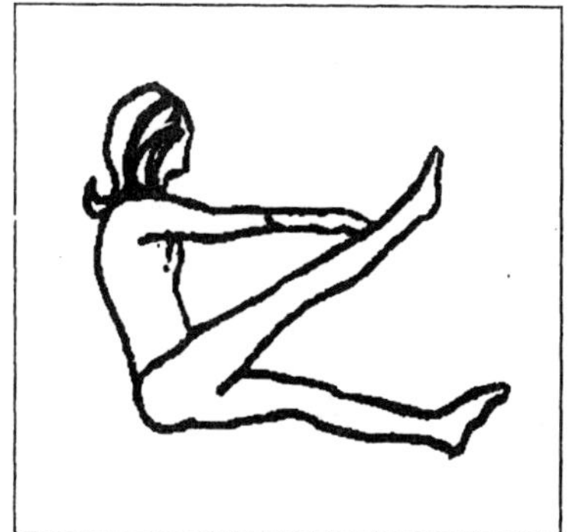

(b) The whole exercise should be repeated with the right leg.

Exercises for Arms and Breasts

1. *(i)* Stand erect. Extend both the arms straight over the head. The palms should be pointing towards the back.

   (ii) Now, turn the palms towards front. Bring the hands down in line with the shoulders.

   (iii) Now raise the arms over the head with palms in front.

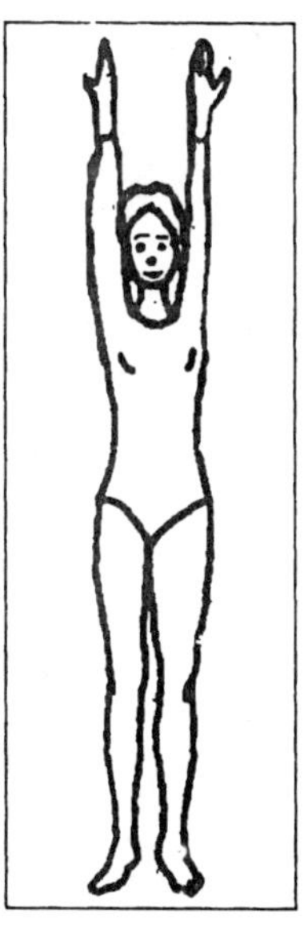

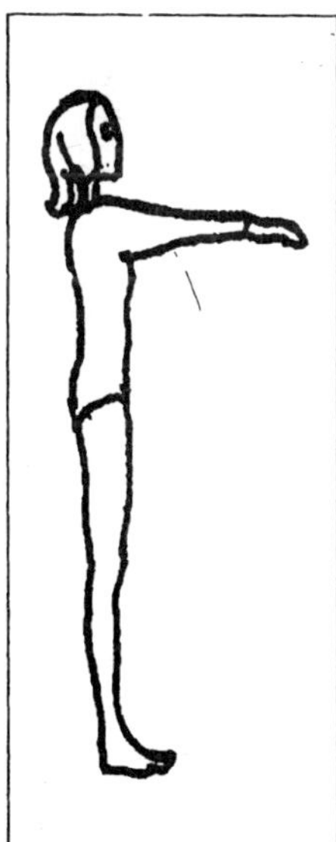

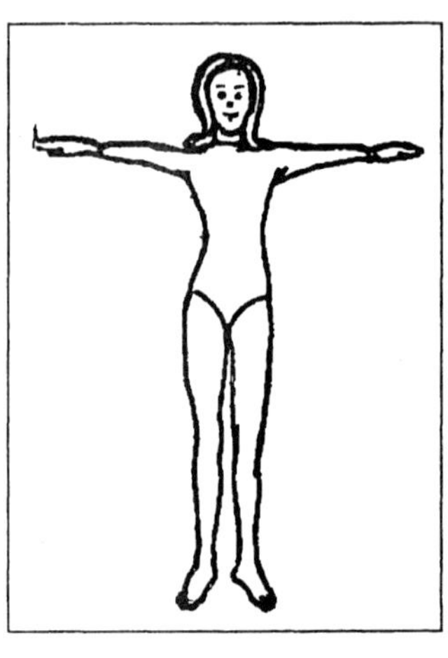

(iv) Turn the palms upwards and bring down the arms in line with the shoulders. This completes the exercise.

Repeat this exercise fifteen times.

2. *(a)* *Stand erect.* Extend both the arms in front of you in line with your shoulders. Join the palms together:

Extend the arms outwards with palms point towards the ground. The arms should remain in line with the shoulders. Palms should be in the direction of the ground.

(b) *Stand erect.* Extend both the arms in front and in line with the shoulders. Join the back of the one hand with the back of the other hand.

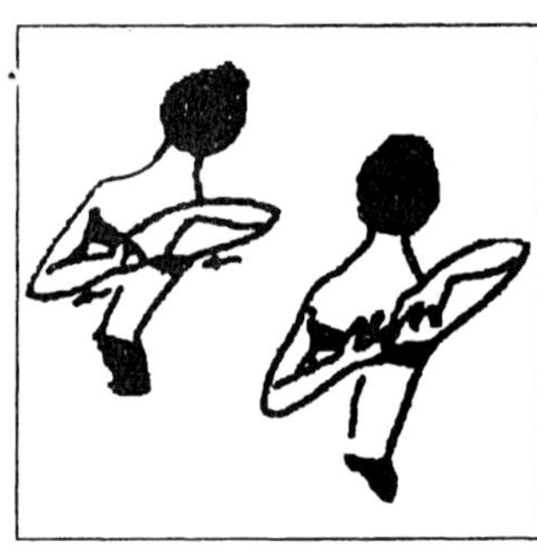

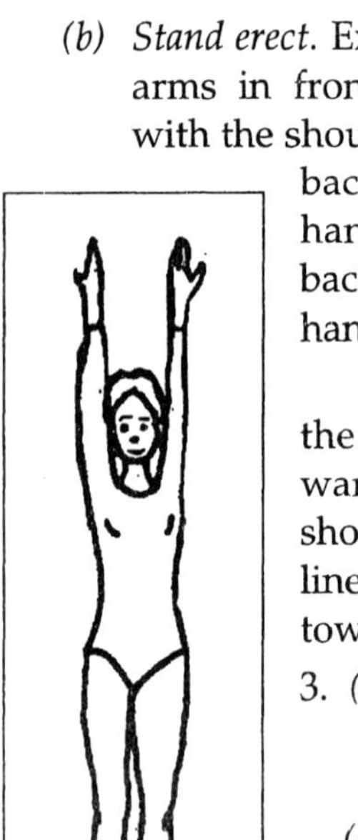

Extend both the arms outwards. The palms should face the ceiling. The arms should be in line with the shoulders, with palms pointing towards the ceiling.

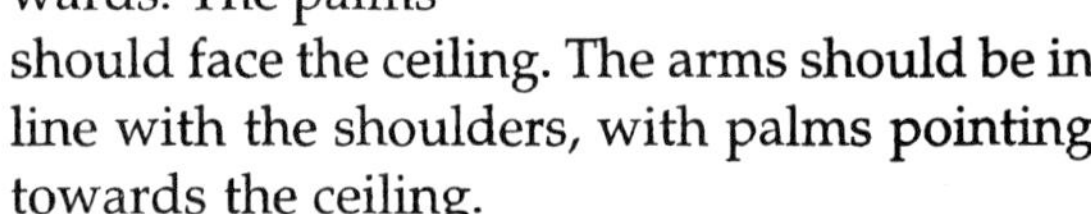

3. *(i)* *Stand erect.* Extend both the arms sideways. The palms should face the ground.

(ii) Now take the arms towards the back and stretch them out-wards to the maximum limit. Remember the arms should re- main straight in the line of shoulders.

(iii) Flex the arms in front ten times.

(iv) Now take them back ten times

Special instructions: Now we shall tell you about the exercises to strengthen the upper part of the arms and the body. You should have dumb-bells for doing these exercises. Each dumb-bell should weight one kilogram. If you do not have dumb-bells these exercises can be performed with weights, thick books, brass tumblers etc. in your hands. It would be better if you buy dumb-bells from any sports shop.

4. Stand erect and then bend the body from the waist. You should have dumb-bells in your hands. They should be held lengthwise as shown in the illustration. The back should remain straight and the abdomen should be drawn inside. Dumb-bells should be held in the manner that the palms face each other. Now, straighten your body and extend the arms sideways in line with the shoulders. Then, again bend at the waist and bring the arms down. This exercise should be repeated ten times.

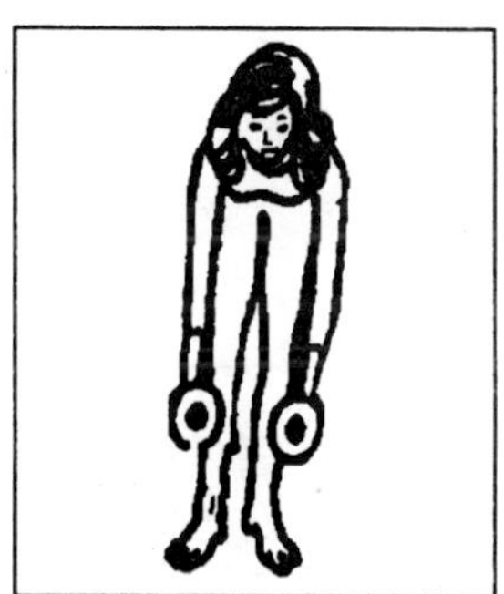

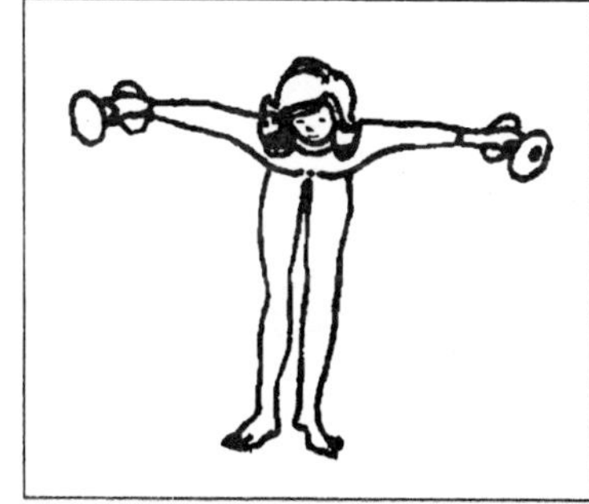

5. Lie on your back. The legs should touch the ground. Now, bend the knees. They should touch each other. The dumb-bells should be in your hands. Take both the arms in the opposite direction over your chest to form a scissor. Take care that the arms are straight and do not bend at any point. Then, extend the arms sideways (right-left) so that they

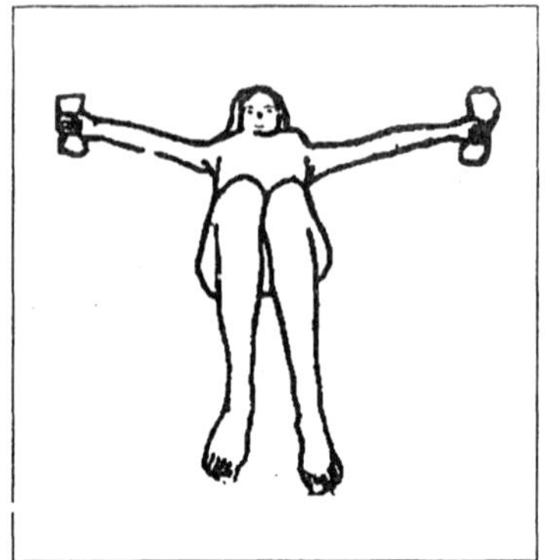

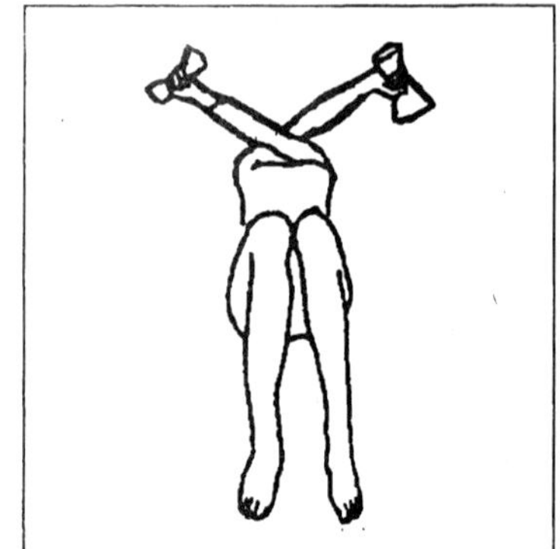

touch the ground. This exercise should also be repeated ten times.

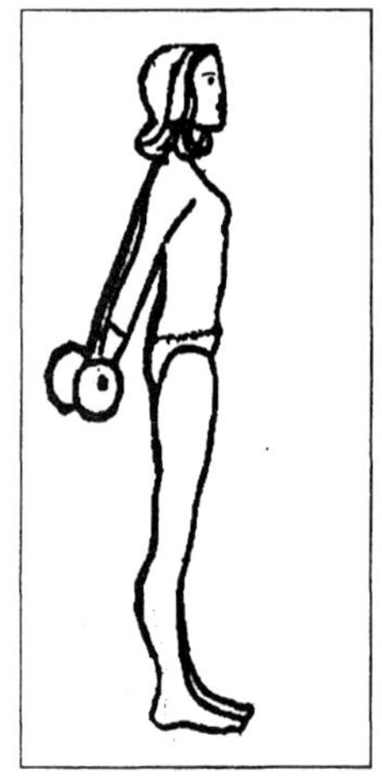

6. (a) *Stand erect.* Hold dumb-bells in your hands. Take the arms backwards.

Touch the ends of dumb-bells with each other. Now extend your arms upwards ten times. The arms should be absolutely straight and the palms should face the sky.

(b) Again extend your arms upwards, taking care that they are straight. This time the palms should face the ground.

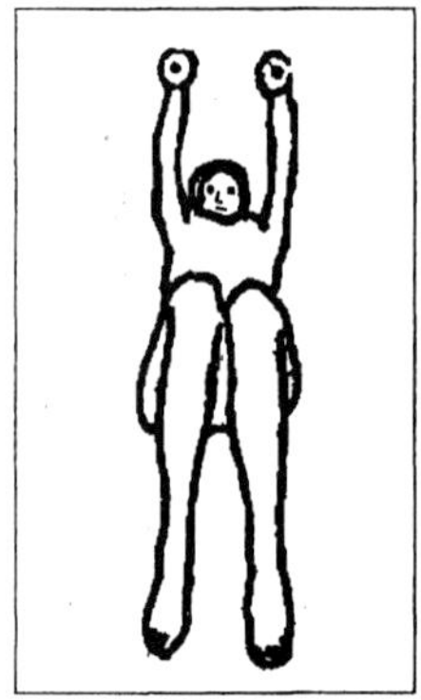

7. (a) Lie on your back. The legs should be bent and the knees should touch each other. Hold dumb-bells in your hands. Extend the arms sideways. The palms should be towards the sky. The arms should not touch the ground. Bring both the arms up so that the palins face each other. Repeat it ten times.

(b) The above exercise should again be done ten times. But, this time while extending the arms upwards, the back of the hands should face each other.

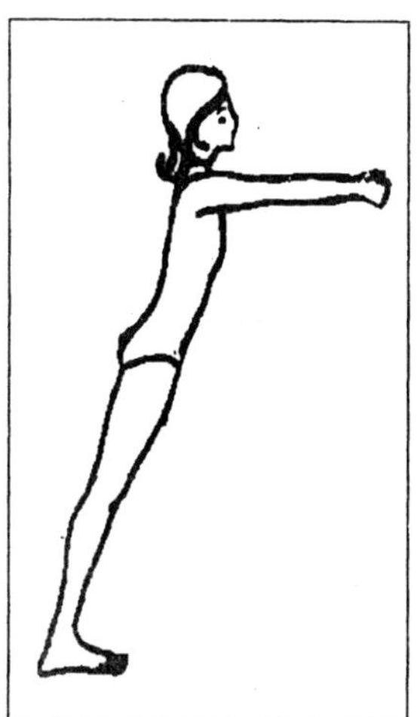

8. *(a)* Stand facing a wall. The distance between the wall and your body should be about 30 Cm. Extend the arms in front of you. Rest your palms on the wall. The fingers of your hand should face each other and should be 15 Cm. away from each other. The' back should be straight and the heels firmly placed on the ground.

   (b) Bend the upper por of your body and place your hands on the wall. Put as much pressure as you can, as if you are trying to push away the wall. Let the elbows also bend. Your chest should touch the wall when you bend. Then, straighten the arms and resume position *(a)*. Repeat this exercise ten times.

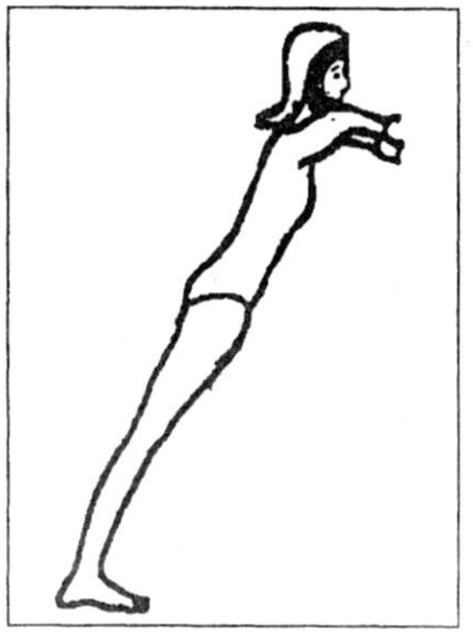

9. *(a)* Lie on your back. Bend your legs. The knees should touch each other. The feet should rest on the ground. Take the dumb-bells in your hands. Bring both your arms parallel to your body. The hands should not touch the ground. They should be in a slightly raised position. Now take both the

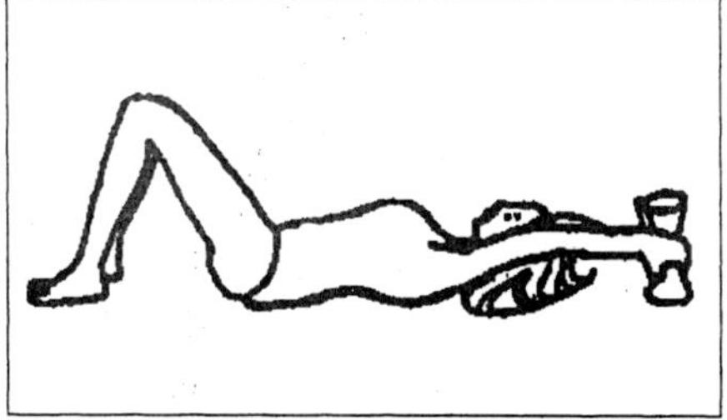

arms over your head. The palms should point outwards. The dumbbells should rest on the ground. Repeat it ten times.

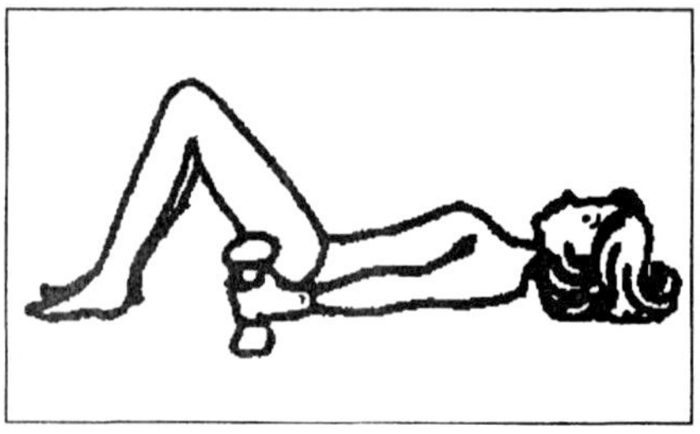

(b) Repeat as in *(a)*. This time the palms should face each other when you take your arms over your head. Do this ten times

Exercises for Hips and Thighs

1. *(a)* Lie on the ground supporting yourself with your arms. The knees should be bent to support your body. Raise your left leg high in the air with the sole facing the ground.

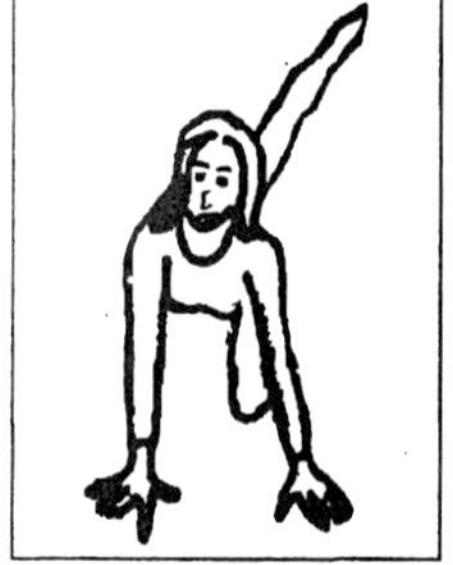

Now, move the extended leg towards the left side. Then bring it towards your back. Repeat this ten times.

(b) Now do the above exercise ten times with your right leg.

2. *(a)* Extend your left leg towards left. The feet should then rest on the ground. Then again lift the leg and put it on the ground. Repeat this ten times.

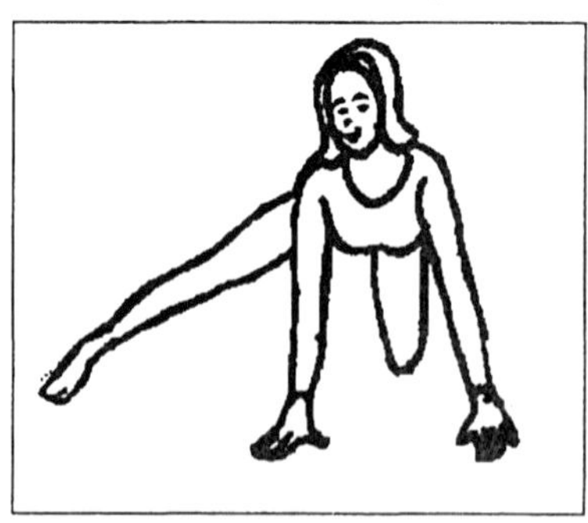

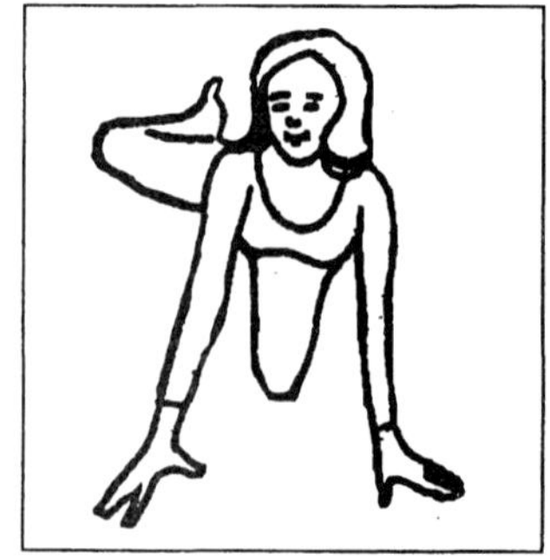

(b) Now do the same exercise with your right leg as detailed in *(a)*. Repeat this ten times.

3. *(a)* Raise your left leg parallel to your hips. The knee should be in a bent position. The ankle should be a little lower. Keep the leg loose. Now extend the left leg towards the left and then bring it back to the original straight position. Repeat this exercise ten times.

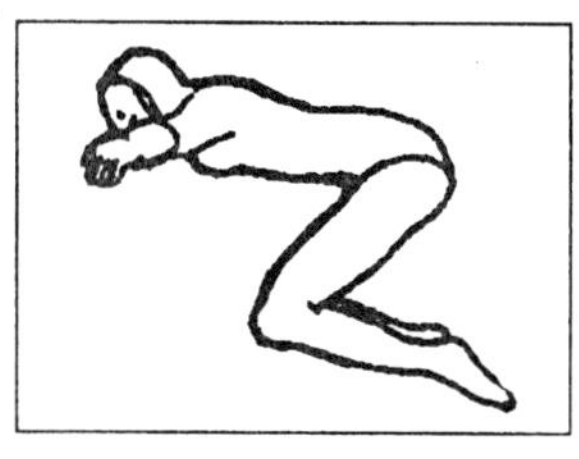

   (b) Now do this exercise in the same manner With your right leg. Repeat it ten times.

4. *(a)* Extend your left leg fully towards the left. Then, sit on your heels. Resume the original position. Then, again extend the leg towards left. Do it five times.

   (b) Repeat the above exercise five times with the right leg.

5. *(a)* Rest your body on your left arm and lie on your left side. The left leg underneath should be a little bent. Take your right leg towards your backside and then bring it in front. Do this exercise ten times. Remember your feet should remain still.

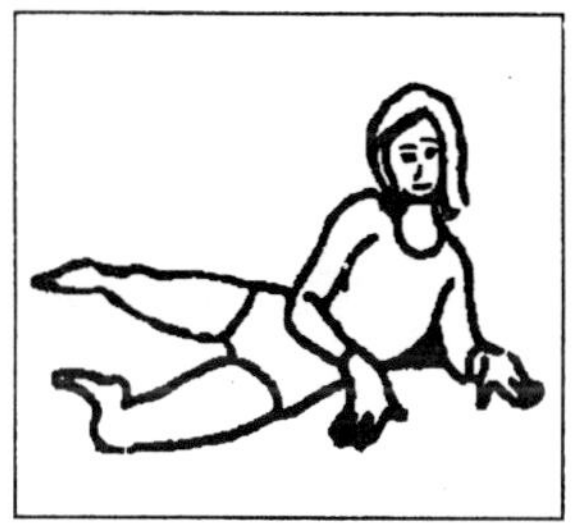

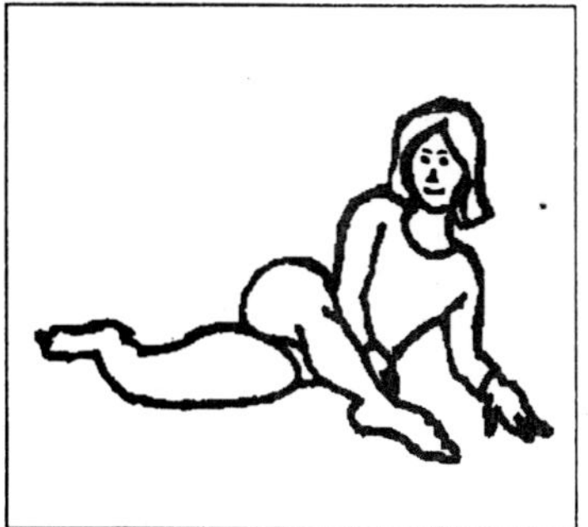

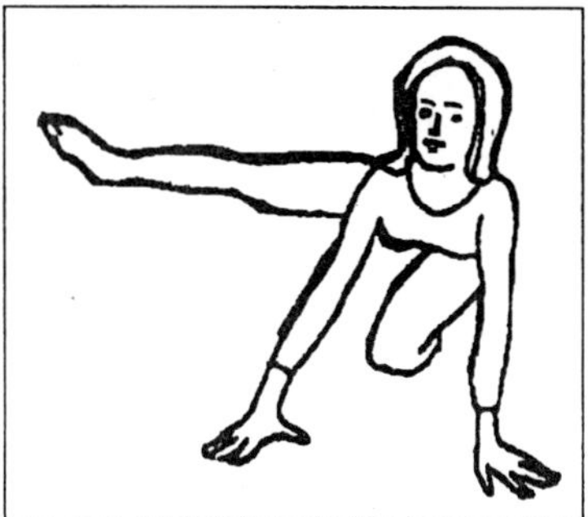

(b) The above exercise *(a)* should now be repeated by lying on the right side on the right arm. Now, do it with your left leg. Repeat it ten times.

6. *(a)* *(i)* Lie on your left side resting your body on the elbow. Keep the right arm on the ground. The body should be straight. The left shoulder, left hip and left knee should be in a straight line. The left leg which is underneath should be slightly bent. The knee of the upper right leg should face the ground. The heels should point towards the sky. Now lift the right leg as much as you can. Then, bring it down and raise again. Repeat it twenty times.

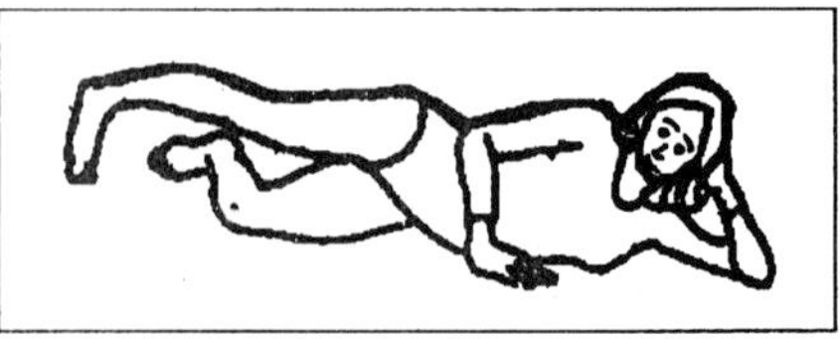

(ii) Now raise your body a little resting on both the arms and repeat the exercise explained in *(a)*.

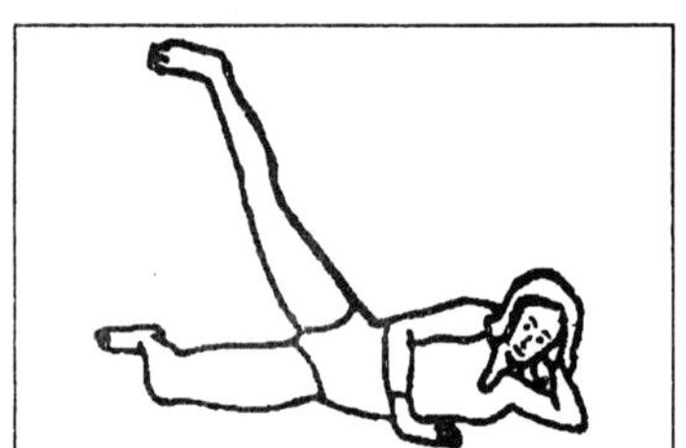

(b) Now do the above exercise, enumerated in *(a)* *(i)* and *(ii)*, lying on your right side. This time the left leg should be raised. Repeat it twenty times.

1. *(a)* Stand erect facing a wall. Extend both your arms in front. Rest your hands on the wall. The fingers should point towards the sky. Your waist should be parallel to the wall. The back should be absolutely straight. Extend your left leg towards the back side. The feet should be about 2 inches

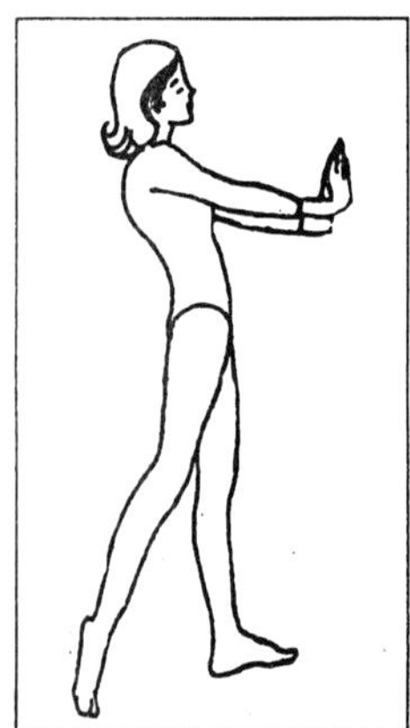

above the ground. Now bring the leg up in a curve. The knee should not bend as far as possible. Repeat it ten times. Now do this exercise ten times again. This time bend the knee.

(*b*) Now do the above exercise (*a*) with the right leg.

Remember: While doing the above exercise, take care that your hips remain straight. They should not bend towards the back. You should make all efforts to prevent this.

2. Lie on the ground on your abdomen. Raise your legs and arms up simultaneously. Neither the elbows nor the knees should bend. Remain in this position for a few seconds. Now move the legs slowly as you do while swimming. Repeat it ten times. Rest for a few seconds. Then repeat it another ten times.

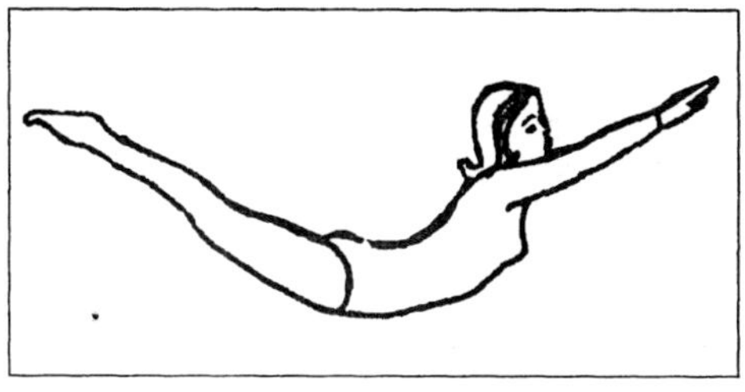

Now relax yourself. This entire exercise should be done thrice. A rest of few seconds should be taken in between.

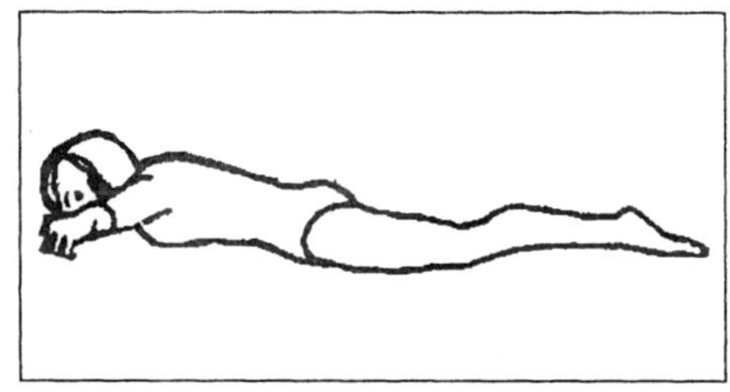

3. Use a strong desk or table for this exercise. Lie on the table on your abdomen. The waist should be on the edge of the table. The table should be narrow in breadth so that you can hold its sides firmly. Bring your knees under the table. The lower portion of your legs upto the knees should be parallel to the ground. Join both the legs and feet together in this position. Now extend your legs backwards and try to take them as high as you can. Come back to the original position. Repeat it ten times.

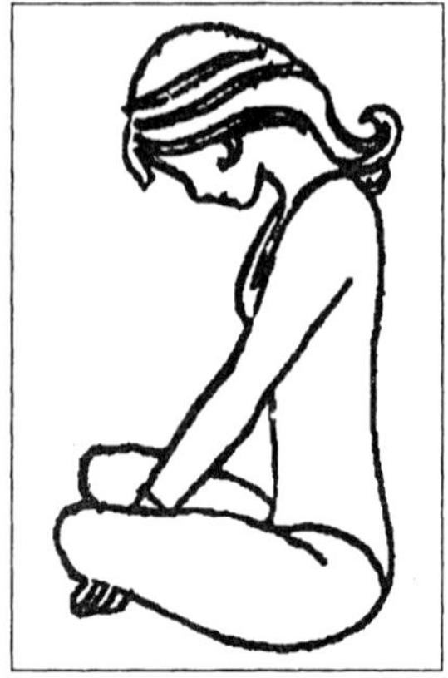

Sit cross-legged on the ground. Draw your stomach inside. Bend the neck downwards and remain in the resting position.

Now, take your head back. Keep the neck as straight as possible. Open your mouth so .that your head is tilted more towards your shoulders. Close the mouth. Remain in this position for ten seconds. Repeat the exercise ten times. This exercise has to be done regularly for reducing the excess fat on the neck and jaws. They will become more shapely.

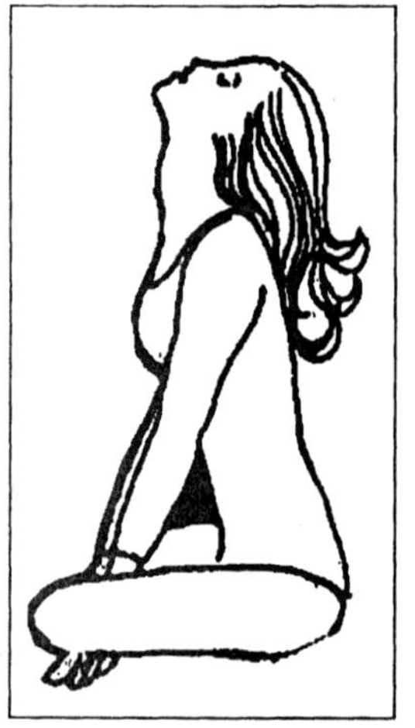

(a) Lie on your back. Bend your legs from the knees. The knees should be in a touching position. The feet should be firmly on the ground. Raise your back and waist slowly so that your entire weight is on your shoulders. Repeat it ten times.

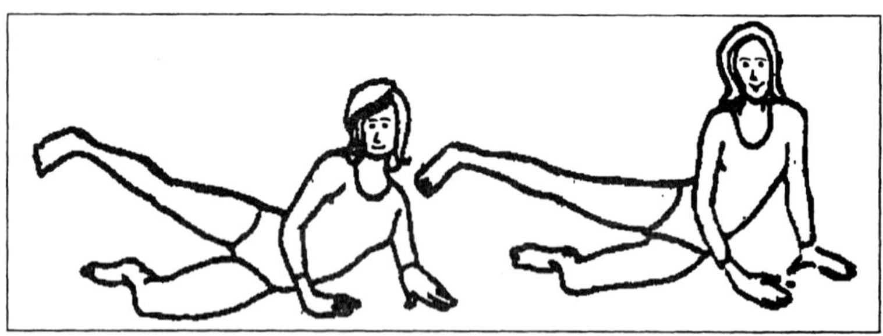

(b) When you are in the position (A), slowly turn your neck towards right and left.

Now, slowly lower your body so that each nerve of your spinal column touches the ground one-by-one. Thereafter, lie straight on the ground.

Repeat this exercise till you feel completely relaxed and the tiredness of your body dispppears.

This exercise should be done after you feel tired from the day's work. It would also be done when your are tired from doing exercises. It removes the tightness of the neck. The back feels rested and the entire body is relaxed.

■

19

Physical Exercises to Shed Weight

There are several physical exercises which can be helpful in increasing your height. Here I have discussed some of these exercises.

Cycling: Stationary and Road

Caloric expenditure during cycling depends more on mechanical gears and the terrain, than on actual distance travelled. Therefore, instead of outlining specific distances and time(as in the Running fitness Progression) the Cycling Programme simply requires that to keep your heart rate in the training zone (70-85%) mhr) for specific amounts of time.

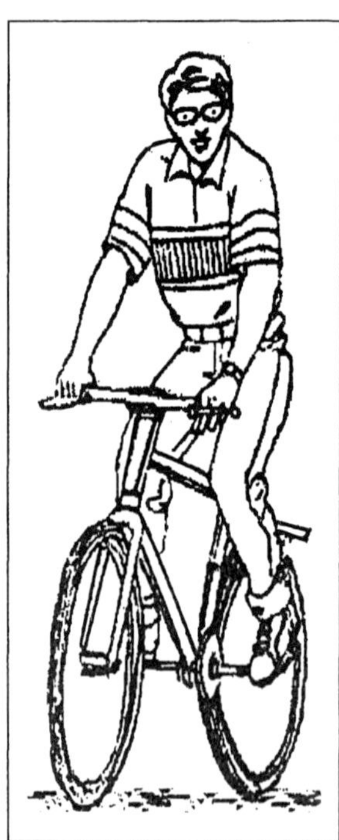

On a stationary bicycle, evaluate your exercise heart rate while pedalling.Road cycling involves move skill and balance,so it is necessary to stop completely for the heart rate check. By the time you reach the Maintenance level, your sensations of exertion will give you a reliable measure of your exercise intensity.

If you haven't been on a bicycle for some time, start with the cycling starter Programme. Your thigh muscles perform most of the work in cycling, and a long gradual conditioning is necessary to avoid pain and injury. But once you become conditioned to cycling, the localised muscular action provides excellent leg strength, and will complement other sports like basketball, skiing and tennis.

Most athletic and health clubs have stationary bicycles. For the real enthusiast, home models can be purchased from major department stores for Rs. 2,500-5,000. Be sure the stationary bike you use is well built and has a knob or lever that can increase wheel resistance. Changing wheel resistance is the main way to control exercise intensity. Cycling faster will also increase intensity, But as you become more fit, the sufficiently high pedal speeds necessary at low resistance levels, are hard to maintain.

Stationary Cycling can be very helpful, and a perfect exercise for rainy days. On the other hand, the monotony of cycling in an open place can make it very boring. you can conquer this problem by combining other diverting activities with your cycling.Try talking to a friend;some people watch television; others catch up on their reading.

The cycling Fitness Progression will be easy to follow if you live in a rural area. The point is to try and keep the cycling pace continuous and consistent. If there are breaks, only count the time spent cycling above 70% MHR. Sometimes it will take a 30-40 minute ride to achieve 20 minutes of real exercise. Remember, coasting downhill is fun, but dies not improve cardiovascular fitness or burn extra calories.

Running

The constant 'pounding' active of this sport is stressful to the feet, legs and back, so a gradual introduction is important. That's why the Walk-jog Starter Programme recommends slow jogging for short periods of time. (By definition, a jog utilises running act upon, but propels the body at walking speed 6-8 km per hour) Running speeds of 10 and 11 kmph should be avoided until the Fitness Progression.

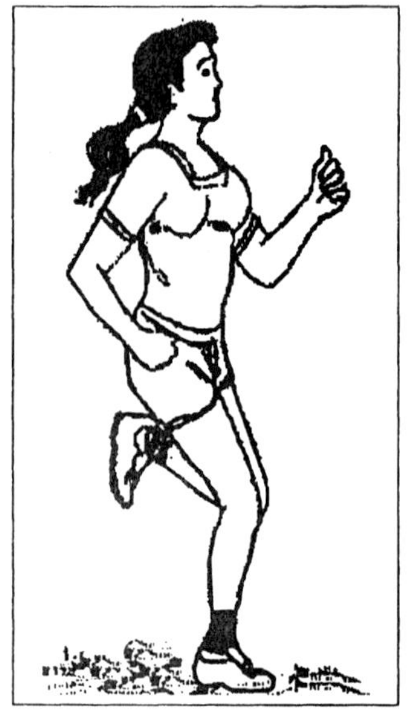

Running is a sport, where doing too much too soon, will cause injury and keep you from becoming a real runner. It is common to feel energetic at the start of a run and to want to burst into high gear.Likewise,many people want to sprint home at the end of a run, with the feeling that they are, somehow,doing something extra towards achieving a high level of fitness. Both actions are foolish; they offer few physical benefits and can be very debilitating to the bones and muscles. A good motto for the runner is 'start slow and taper off at the end'.

Good running shoes are a must, no matter what the price. Tennis shoes or cheap sneakers are the surest way to ruin a running career. Buy your running shoes at a sports shop or athletic shoes store. There are many good brands; select the one that feels most comfortable.

Finally, running is an excellent sport for the heart, but it has a negative effect on flexibility. Leg and back muscles become tight, and if left unattended you can pull the hip and vertebra out of alignment. Moreover, running the next day with stiff muscles is the perfect way to injure them and disable yourself. So be sure to do the Warm-up Routine faithfully before each run. Spend a little extra time stretching the lower back and legs you can get additional relief from muscle tightness by repeating the Warm-up routine after each run and on non- running days.

Swimming

Swimming is a unique sport that has advantages and disadvantages compared to running .On the plus side, swimming provides optimal cardiovascular and weight control benefits without risk of leg injury. Many people who feel awkward and uncomfortable while running find this non-weight-bearing sport delightfully easy. For this same reason, land-bound athletes suffer from hip, knee and ankle problem.

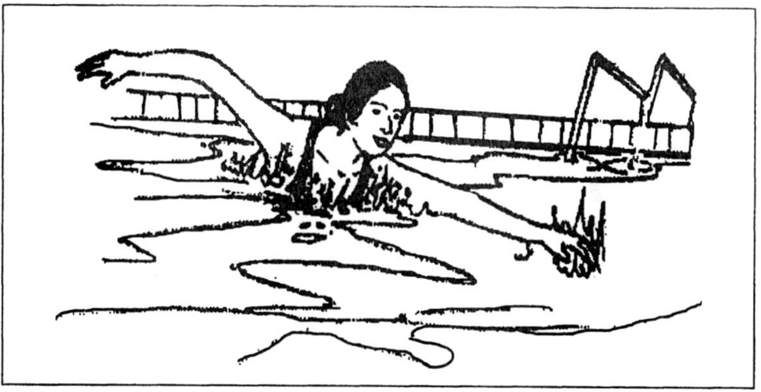

But, Whereas, swimming does wonders for upper body strength, it is not so good for the lower- body (anti-gravity) musculature of the body. Obviously, swimmers don't fall down when they climb out of the pool, but their performance in land sports is definitely compromised by a total swimming programme. On the other hand, a combination of swimming and running makes an excellent programme for all around muscular development.

Breaststroke, backstroke, butterfly, and freestyle are the acceptable swimming strokes for the Progression programme. Side stroke and other floating strokes are less vigorous, and not useful for general conditioning. A proper swimming technique is a must for fitness development as well as sport enjoyment. The caloric cost of the Swimming chart assumes average or good skill level. If you need basic instructions, many fine adult swimming courses are available at sports institutions, YMCA, YWCA, etc.

Measuring exercise heart rate during a swimming workout is possible, but the validity of the results can be questionable. (Some swimmers leave a watch at one end of the pool and check heart rate after swimming two lengths.) Sports scientists discovered years ago that exercise on land. Therefore, the swimming heart rate can, at best, be considered a rough guide of exercise intensity. If a new exercise level feels particularly difficult or leaves you tired for the rest of the day, drop back to the previous level for another week.

Walking

Walking is the number one sport for convenience because it fits nicely into the normal daily routine. Trips to the corner market and a night or after-dinner stroll, all provide good exercise without a lot of fanfare. Sturdy, comfortable shoes that have good arch support, are the only equipment needed.

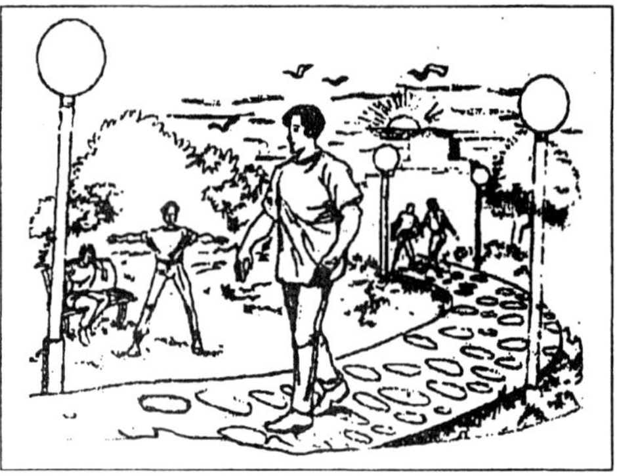

The low caloric cost of walking-3-6 calories per minute, means that exercise duration must be longer than with intensive activity, to expend sufficient energy. Other continuous sports can burn 300 Calories in 30 minutes; with walking, it takes 60-90 minutes. However, you don't have to do it all at once. Separate 15-20 minutes walks throughout the day bring the same results.

Walking is always an excellent exercise for weight control, but the low intensity offers no cardiovascular stimulus for those already in good condition. Walking at 6-7 kmph makes it difficult to elevate your heart rate above the minimum 70% MHR. For this reason, the running programme is generally recommended; but if walking is your joy, here are two suggestions for increasing exercise intensity:

1. Find a long, gradually sloping hill to walk up.
2. Carry a small pack on your back and add whatever weight is necessary to keep your exercise heart rate at 70-85% MHR.

There is no starter programme for the walking, everyone begins at Level I using a high track and a watch, you can get a good feeling for the different walking speeds (two laps around the standard track equal 800 metres). You can also plot your own measured distance by driving over the route you select, and checking the distance on the odometer. In addition, you can check your local sporting goods store for pedometers—devices which you can clip to your belt to count footsteps and calculate distance walked. Pedometers cost Rs. 450-600.

Rope Skipping and Stationary Running

Exercises certainly stimulate the cardiovascular system, but they are very hard on the feet, ankles and lower leg muscles. With walking and running, the foot lands-heel first, and the strong, straightened, long leg bones absorb the shock. But during hopping, the ball of the foot takes the initial shock and then transmits the stress to injury-prone ankles and lower leg muscles. This makes hopping exercises very hazardous.

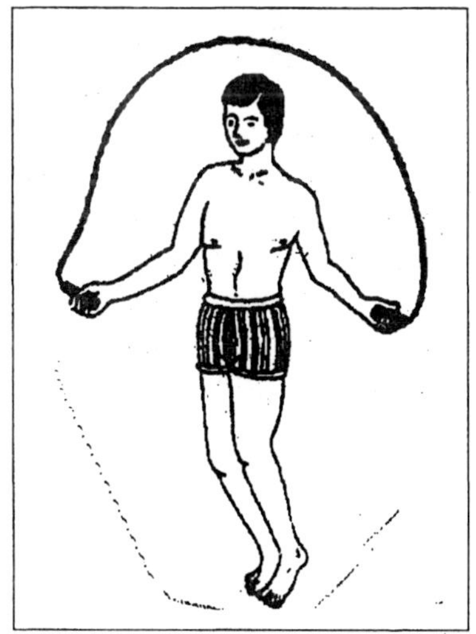

Uncontrollable exercise intensity is another problem with rope skipping and stationary running. (To hop more slowly, you have to jump higher to maintain rhythm; this requires approximately the same energy as short jumps at a quicker pace. So it is very difficult to develop a programme of graduated intensity.)

Therefore, rope skipping and stationary running are not generally recommended. (Competitive athletes may use these exercises for conditioning, but only with a carefully designed programme of interval training: alternate periods of hopping and rest, slowly building up a total workout time of 20-30 minutes).

Stair Climbing and Bench Stepping

Stair climbing and bench stepping are the recommended home exercises for most people. The stress on feet, ankles and knees is greater than with walking, but still well below that of rope skipping and stationary running. Most important, however, the intensity of exercise can be precisely controlled through adjustments in bench height and stepping rate.

Stair climbing can provide adequate exercise with appropriate adjustment of climbing rate to reach the 70-85% MHR training zone. You start with one minute of continual climbing the first week, and add one minute each week thereafter (exercise 3-4 days a week); final maintenance level is 20-30 minutes of continual climbing.

If stairs are not available, a 24-30 cm. stepping bench can be used. If you decide to construct such a bench, be sure it is well made and holds firm even on slippery floors. Follow the progression guidelines for stair climbing. The correct technique involves four steps: left foot up, right foot up left foot down, right foot down. It's all right to.hold on to a nearby rail for balance, but do not pull yourself up on the bench: make the leg muscles perform all the work.

■

5-Week Cycling Starter Programme (Road or Stationary)

	Cycling Days per Week	Intensity Time (min.) per session	Rest Time (min.) (% MHR)	Repeat between cycling sessions	Total cycling cycling Time sessions	+ Rest (min.)
1st Week	3	2	70%	2	Twice	6
2nd Week	3	3	70%	3	Twice	9
3rd Week	4	4	70%	3	Twice	11
4th Week	4	5	70%	2	Twice	12
5th Week	4	6	70%	1	Twice	13

Cycling Progression Programme
(Road or Stationary)

Level	Intensity (% MHR)	Total Time, Each Session (min.)
I	70-85%	13
II	70-85%	14
III	70-85%	15
IV	70-85%	16
V	70-85%	17
VI	70-85%	18
VII	70-85%	19
VIII	70-85%	20
Maintenance	70-85%	20-30

Minimum Progression
(Exercise 3-4 days a week)

		Caloric Cost	
Age	**Exercise Days At each level**	**Weight Kg**	**Calories per min. at 20 kmph**
Below 30	4	57	9.0
30-39	6	68	10.9
40-49	8	80	12.7
50 and above	11	90	14.6

Running

Level	Fast walk Time (min)	Distance (in kms)	Run Time (min)	Repetitions	Total Time (min)
I	4	0.8	6	2	20
II	6	1.6	11	1	17
III	7	1.6	10	1	17
IV	5	2.4	15	1	20
V	5	2.4	14	1	19
VI	1	3.2	19	1	20
VII	1	3.2	18	1	19
VIII		4.0	22	1	22
Main-tenance		4-6.4	20-35	1	20-35

Minimum Progression (Exercise 3-4 days a week)

		Caloric Cost	
Age	**Exercise Days At each level**	**Weight Kg**	**Calories per min. at 10.0 kmph to 13.0 kmph**
Below 30	4	57	12.1
30-39	6	68	14.5
40-49	8	80	16.9
50 and above	11	90	19.3

Swimming
(Road or Stationary)

Level	Distance (min.)	Total Time (min.)
I	270	9
II	270	8
III	360	10
IV	450	13
V	540	15
VI	630	18
VII	720	20
VIII	810	23
Maintenance	900-1350	20-40

Minimum Progression
(Exercise 3-4 days a week)

		Caloric Cost		
	Exercise Days	Weight	Calories per min. at	
Age	At each level	Kg	36 m./min	45 m./min
Below 30	4	57	8.0	8.9
30-39	6	68	9.7	10.8
40-49	8	80	11.4	12.6
50 and above	11	90	13.1	14.5

5-Week Swimming Starter Programme
(Road or Stationary)

	Swimming Days per Week	Swimming Time (min.) per session	Swimming Distance (mrt)	Rest Time between Swimming sessions	Repeat Swimming sessions	Total Swimming + Rest Time (min.)
1st Week	3	1.5	45	3	2	6
2nd Week	3	1.5	45	2	3	8.5
3rd Week	4	3.0	90	2	2	8
4th Week	4	5.0	135	1	2	11
5th Week	4	4.5	135	1	2	10

Walking

Level	Distance (km.)	Speed (kmph)	Total Time (min)
I	1.0	3.0	20
II	1.5	3.0	30
III	1.5	3.25	28
IV	2.0	3.25	38
V	2.0	3.5	35
VI	2.5	3.5	43
VII	3.0	3.5	50
VIII	3.25	3.5	55
Maintenance	3.5-4.5	3.5	60-80

Minimum Progression (Exercise 3-4 days a week)

		Caloric Cost		
	Exercise Days	Weight	Calories per min. at	
Age	At each level	Kg	36 m./min	45 m./min
Below 30	4	57	3.0	3.5
30-39	6	68	3.6	4.2
40-49	8	80	4.2	4.9
50 and above	11	90	4.8	5.6

20

What to Do, if Exercise and Dieting Do Not Prove Efficacious?

If you feel that dieting and exercises are not proving efficacious at a rapid pace, specially if the fat on your abdomen and hips is not diminishing, you can adopt a special bath that would definitely prove helpful in reducing the unwanted fat on the abdomenal region. This special method of taking bath is known as 'Hip bath'

Method—For taking this bath a tub is used which has a backrest. Such tubs are available in the market.

In case, you are unable to buy such a tub, you can use any circular tub used for washing clothes. You can rest your back against the wall.

Fill the tub with clear cold water upto three-fourth of its height. The tub should be placed near the wall so that you can easily rest your back against the wall when you sit in the tub.

Now, take off your clothes and sit in the tub wearing only an underwear. Your back will rest against the wall and legs should be out of the tub upto your thighs. It is advisable to keep your feet on a wooden plank rather than on the ground. In this position, your abdomen, waist and hips will be submerged in the water of the tub. Remember, the water in the tub should be upto a level so that your navel is out of water.

Now, loosen your abdomen. After sitting in this position for two minutes, take a soft cloth or towel and rub your body, below the navel, and from right to left. This massage should start from the right side of your waist to the left side without lifting the cloth or the towel. Do not rub with force. If you do so, you may feel a burning sensation or the skin might be bruised. Continue this procedure for some time and then come out and dry your body.

On the 1st day take this bath for ten minutes. Then gradually increase its duration taking 20-25 minutes everyday.

You will find remarkable change in the size of your waist and hips within a week. The fat on the abdomen and hips will start vanishing and your weight will be reduced by one-and-a-half to two kilograms. In case, you find your weight going down too much in two days, do not take up bath daily. Do it on alternate days, or even twice a week. Hip bath usually has instant effect.

When to take Hip Bath

If you wish to include hip bath along with exercises and dieting, then do it before the exercises and breakfast. Exercises and breakfast should be after the bath. Hip bath is very efficacious on an empty stomach.

During summer use cold water and in winter use luke-warm water. During winter hip bath should be taken in a closed room, otherwise it may prove harmful.

We have mentioned about the hip bath separately as it should be adopted only when exercises and dieting do not prove very effective. Hip bath is an excellent device to reduce sagging abdomen and hips to normal size, particularly after child-birth.

For dieting, we have prescribed expensive as well as inexpensive diets. You can choose any according to your taste. All the diets are based on authentic research and recommended by the doctors.

Another important point is that you need not unduly worry about your weight or flabby body. Worry has harmful effect on your body and even affects your mind. Do your exercises with a calm mind. The result will speak for itself.

■

Dieting Chart

DIETING CHART COURSE NO. 1

Your diet to reduce your weight and fatness

About 1200 calories

On getting up in the morning: Juice of lemon in cold or hot water. Tea without sugar.

Breakfast

Toned Milk	8 oz. (one glass)
Bread	2 slices
Dalia	1 oz.
Corn Flakes	1 oz.

In between breakfast and lunch—(If you take your lunch late)

Tea or coffee or fruit juice (without sugar)

Lunch

Flou	3 small chapatis or
Rice	2 oz.
Pulses	1½
Curd	6 oz. or
Cheese	2 oz. or
Meat, fish or chicken	4 oz.
Vegetables	as much as you like.

Afternoon

Tea, or coffee or fruit juice (without sugar)	
Salted Biscuits	3 or
Cream Crackers	2

Dinner

Similar to lunch

Ghee or oil 2 teaspoonfuls (for the whole day)

Prohibited Food

1. Full cream milk, cream, butter, oil, ghee and fried articles, gur.
2. Sugar,bura, honey and sweets of all kinds.
3. Ovaltine, horlicks, coco etc.
4. Banana, mangoes ahd grapes.
5. Potato, gentleman's toe (arvi) and 'zaminkand'.
6. Coca cola and cold drinks.
7. Wine.

Proposed Diets

1. Vegetables, tomato, kheera, radish, lemon, vegetable or mutton soup, lassi, pickles, chatni, zeera jal and amla.
2. Tea or coffee (without sugar).
3. Toned milk and articles made therefrom.

Note: If you like, you may take sacrine in place of sugar. If you suffer from high blood pressure along with fatness, you should not take salt, soda and sacrine.

DIETING CHART COURSE NO. 2

1,200 calories **Vegetarian/non-vegetarian**

Break Fast

Egg	1 (not fried) 25 grams

(or cheese)	
Toned milk	240 ml
Bread	50 grams
Tea	1 Cup
Lunch	
Pulses	50 grams
Seasonal vegetables (cooked)	375 grams
Curd	100 grams
Chapati	100 grams
Boiled rice	100 grams
Dinner	
Meat, fish or chicken	50 grams or
Cheese or grams	25 grams
Cooked vegetables	375 grams
Chapati	100 grams
Rice	100 grams

■

22

Diet Therapy with Ideal Menu

We all eat to live but a balanced diet is must for a long life. For diseases, the diet should be consulted by an expert.

Detoxification Diet

Fruit, raw vegetables, youghurt and water are recommended to eliminate toxins that are caused by poor digestion of waste products absorbed from the environment. Allergies, arthritis are claimed to be allayed by detoxification process.

Raw Food Diet

It was developed by a swiss doctor. It consists of 70% of raw fruit and vegetables, 30% grains, dairy products, meat and nuts. It improves digestion and increases longevity and is said to maintain food's chemical activity due to its being taken in cooked form.

Vegetarian Diet

Only meat and fish are excluded but dairy products and eggs are included in it. Apart from inclusion of major portion of vegetables and fruits. Vegetarianism is said to reduce risk of high blood pressure, diabetes, heart disease, cancer of colon and osteoporosis. Vegetarian diet is being accepted as an all inclusive potent food plan toward many health problems.

Microbiotic Diet

This diet was intorduced by George Osawa, a Japanese practitioner who chose certain food items which stood the test of Yin or Yang factors. Foods like fruits, nuts and vegetables are called calming foods and this, nomenclated as 'Yin foods' whereas root vegetables, cereals and fish are called strengthening foods or 'Yang foods'

Gerson Therapy

This goods therapy devised by an American doctor Dr. Max Gerson who described it as an anti-cancer regime. It aims at raising the alkaline level of body tissues. It is based on organic vegie diet, low salt, supplemented with an hourly intake of vegetable and fruit juice and coffee enemas. It is a controversial therapy, having no medical and therapeutical support,.

Vegan Diet

This dietary pattern excludes eggs, dairy products and honey but realise only on fruits and vegetables. This diet is deficient in Vitamin B-12. It is a protein enriched diet which is supplied by pulses, grains, nuts and cereals. Disorders like high blood pressure, arthritis, angina, rheumatoid arthritis, asthma are claimed to have been cured by this therapy.

Hay Diet

Dr. William Hay of the United States developed this dietary pattern which is also called a 'Food combining diet.' He was firmly of the view that carbohydrates and proteins should not be taken in the same meals as both of them are the foods that fight. Proteins cause the stomach to produce acid while carbohydrates ought to be digested in alkaline environment, but natural foods can efficiently combine with either group. Hence it is better to eat only Hay diet.

Ornish Reversal Diet

Dr. Deam Ornish believed that an ideal diet should consists of high carbohydrates and fibre, but low in fat and cholesterol but excluding animal products, non fat milk and yoghurt. Some American doctors rely on his suggetions to reverse heart disease, of course with the support of meditation, yoga and exercise.

Indian Diet

Most of our regional diets are generally well-balanced and a person does not have to spend any extra money. In northern India wheat, black gram, pulses, purified ghee, milk yoghurt, whey, raw and cooked vegetables, seasonal fruits form our essential part of the daily diet. Even though most people were not aware of the nutrients i.e. even then their daily diet didn't lack in essential nutrients. Apart from this, vegetations were not toxified by chemical manure, pesticides and insecticides and people inhaled fresh air, moved freely in open fields, exerted their bodies to strenuous activity, took full rest and enjoyed life.

Medium of cooking changed from purified ghee to mustard oil, coconut oil, saffola etc. but milk and milk products were used in one form or the other. People believed in taking 'Satvik food' but in coastal areas sea foods were used may be due to weather demands. Some people lived only on seasonal fruits and milk, whey and curd and maintained normal health.

Foods to be replaced/limited

- Limit intake of cheese and red-meats that are high in saturated fat content.
- Number of calories, obtained from fat, must be kept below 30% of total daily dietary intake of calories.
- Not more than 10% of total fat calories should be obtained of from saturated fat intake.
- Avoid processed and junk foods that are overloaded with flavouring preservatives and colourings.
- Butter should be replaced with soft margarine or low fat foods that are high in polyunsaturated fats. Spread it thinly.
- To keep the blood sugar level within normal confines, consume sugar in limited quantity.
- Salt intake must be limited. Avoid eating salty foods, and also adding (extra) salt to meals. Also do not consume processed meats and crispy eatables.

- Limit use of tea, coffee, cold drinks, chocolates and sweets so as to reduce intake of caffeine, Instead you may use herbal teas with advantage but without hassles.
- Excessive intake of alcohol must be reduced.
- Do not use strong spices and condiments as they irritate stomach.

Ideal Menu and Timings

- On rising early in the morning, drink a glass or two of normal water.
- Take a glass of juice (carrot/apple with sweet lime/orange) before going for a brisk walk around 7.00 a.m. (during summer 6.00 a.m.). May take a cup of skimmed milk after vigorous yogic exercises, if suits.

• *Lunch (10:00 a.m.)* Take nutritious food as you need enough energy for working whole day.	Take good Salad (consume first), cooked vegetables 2 or 3 cups, medium chapati 2-3 or rice 2 cups, 2 cups cooked pulse, 1 or 2 cups of youghurt (Dahi), steamed vegetables 1/2 or 1 cup.
• *Supper (Around 7:00) p.m.)* Out of total 1600 Calories consumed during the whole day, evening meal should not contain more than 350 calories.	As per your taste and chioce but light, e.g. (A) 1 or 2 cooked vegetables, with 1 chapati, and 1 cup of yoghurt or (B) 1 cup soup, I fruit and raw vegetables or (C) 2 cups of skimmed milk with 1 or 2 bananas or apples or toast or bread slices.

If you have to go out for dinner, take just a cup of skimmed milk or soup or eat some roasted grams or some fruits/vegetables at around 6:00 p.m. before going. If you take a late evening dinner, drink a glass of lemon juice (juice of 1 lemon in one glass of warm water) the following morning (empty stomach).

Herbs and Spices

- You may use asafoetida (Hing), cloves, corriander, garlic, ginger, saunf, turmeric, cumin (Jeera), cardamon, ajwain, pepper, and kali rai.
- Bed tea/coffee is very harmful. Avoid tea/coffee/cold drinks and fried items always.

■

23

A Six Week Course for Ladies to Reduce Fat and Weight

We must make it clear in the very beginning that if you adopt this course only for a few weeks to reduce ugly fat and weight and then forget about it, it will be of no use. You have to be careful about your weight for all the time. Often, people who undergo a slimming course complain that their weight went down in the beginning, but it again increased after some time and in the end they found themselves at the same point from which they started.

You must understand the reason for this. The main reason is that usually people are unable to change their habits. It is all the more true regarding dietary habits. You have to firmly resolve that you have to get rid of your obesity and excess weight, then only you can bring about remarkable changes in your habits. It is the will that matters.

We do not expect you to leave or give up food. We also do not ask you to take special food. We only ask you to change yourself and your habits, particularly eating habits. You can become 'your own beauty counsellor and set up your own rules' but resolve to follow them.

Dietary Habits

Physiologists and psychologists have reached the conclusion that different people have different eating habits. Not only that they desire food at different times as well. You must have seen people eating sandwiches while watching television. Some keep a packet of biscuits by their side while reading and eating them when doing so. Many are used to eating cashewnuts, groundnuts or biscuits while enjoying a movie. These people have formed a habit of eating while doing something. This creates a craze to have sandwiches or snacks when viewing television, reading or seeing films.

First, you have to resolve to leave this bad habit. A firm determination is needed. Another mistake is that when we are worried over anything. He try to divert our mind from it by eating something. When we behave better or do something good, the parents reward us with sweets. As we grow up, we immediately and inadvert ently think of eating something in case of tensions, unhappiness, worries etc. or when we are sad or tired. We do not pause to think as to what we are doing. It is an automatic action.

We have to first get rid of such habits. You must leam to identify your bad habits. Analyse your conduct, behaviour and routine. Get ready to, bring about revolutionary changes in your habits. If you do need to have some reward, or consolation, try to select some other things than eatables:

Start giving-up your old habits. Gradually you will feel that you are now treading a more pleasant path. You will never desire to return to your old and discarded habits.

It you adopt sensible dietary habits, and follow it rigidly, you will find that your weight is going down rapidly and your body is becoming agile, active and slender.

First Week

The first thing you have to do is to write down ycur weight. Then record your weight every week on the same day, time and place. The best time to weight yourself is in the morning when you have an empty stomach.

In this first week, you have to know and understand points regarding what you eat, when and where?

Your biggest problem would be snacks. You might have the habit of tasting food while cooking. Some of us have the habit of eating some thing when doing household chores like cleaning wheat or rice. Many times you might be taking a few morsels to check if the salt and other condiments are in right proportion. Following are some statements. Read them carefully and put A, B, or C after them. If you are in the habit of frequently doing them, put 'C' against them. If you do so sometimes, 'B' should be put against them and if you do it rarely, put 'A' against them.

For each 'A' marks are = 0

For 'B' the marks are = 5

'C' carries marks = 10.

Note: Make Scoring Charts' for snacks and substantive meals as per models given on following pages. Put 'A', 'B' or 'C' against the questions given therein and add up the points daily. In this way, prepare the score for a whole week.

Snacks

1. Whenever I feel alone in the house, I have snacks to relieve loneliness.
2. When I am in a sad or indifferent mood, I try to divert my mind by having snacks.
3. When I return to my home and if I am tired, I take some snacks to regain lost energy.
4. I generally take snacks when the workload is heavy and or I am under tension. I feel it helps me in concentrating on my work.
5. I have the habit of munching something while watching programmes on television.
6. I have to make or receive a lot of phone calls. I keep some snacks nearby telephone and take them while making calls.
7. Many a time, I feel that my stomach needs filling and I feel uneasy. To relieve myself of that uneasiness I resort to taking snacks.
8. I take snacks to pass time in train, bus or car.
9. I enjoy snacks while seeing a drama or film.

10. If I am angry due to some discussion or quarrel, I take snacks to suppress my anger.

First Week

Habit No.	First Day	Second Day	Third Day	Fourth Day	Fifth Day	Sixth Day	Seventh Day
1	A	A	A	A	B	A	A
2	C	C	B	B	B	B	C
3	C	B	B	A	A	A	A
4	B	A	A	A	A	C	A
5	A	A	B	A	A	A	B
6	B	C	B	B	A	A	A
7	A	A	A	A	A	A	A
8	C	B	C	C	B	A	A
9	B	A	A	C	B	B	A
10	B	B	A	A	B	A	A
Total	50	35	30	30	25	20	15

Note: Make a chart like one given above. You have to fill it honestly everyday during the week. The total of your score everyday should be added and recorded in the chart.

Meals

1. I watch television while taking meals.
2. While cooking, I taste the things to test their quality.
3. While serving meals, I taste everything that I have cooked to find if others would like them.
4. I do not like throwing away food, hence, I myself eat whatever excess food is on the table.
5. I like the appetite-increasing aroma of the food being cooked and feel forced to taste it.
6. I like to have a lot of chutney or tomato sauce with chapaties or bread.
7. I serve myself in a thali, so that I can eat comfortably on an easy chair.

8. I like serving myself more snacks than others.
9. I feel happy if there is a big helping of anything sweet.
10. If some guest arrives, I eat again just to give him company.

Now test yourself.

Remember

For each' A' the score is 0

The score for 'B' is 5

The score for 'C' is 10

Now honestly put' A', 'B' or 'C' after each question and decide regarding habits that you will have to change. Actually, these are the habits that you have to get rid of.

Your aim should be to get the minimum marks in this test. It should be to score 0. Test yourself every week and see your score. When you score 0, you can consider to have passed tlie test. By that time, your weight would be lesser by 11 to 16 kilograms.

First Week

Habit No.	First Day	Second Day	Third Day	Fourth Day	Fifth Day	Sixth Day	Seventh Day
1	C	C	B	B	B	A	B
2	C	B	B	B	A	B	A
3	A	B	B	B	A	A	A
4	A	A	A	B	A	A	A
5	B	B	B	A	A	B	B
6	A	A	A	A	A	B	A
7	B	A	B	B	B	A	A
8	C	B	B	A	C	A	A
9	A	A	A	A	A	A	A
10	C	C	B	B	B	B	B
Total	50	40	35	30	25	20	15

Directions—You have to fill in this chart giving your score as 'A', 'B' or 'C' according to your daily food habits. Be honest to yourself. You have also to keep in mind that you have to improve upon your habits and control them. Also mention if you have eaten more due to some special circumstances or reasons.

Note: This chart will mirror all your harmful habits and help you in getting rid of them.

Second Week

In this week, you have to analyse your eating habits. Make a chart in the beginning of this week. Record in it if you have broken any rule regarding snacks and meals in the previous week. You must record the rule you have broken as well as the day and time at which it was broken. You will have a summary of the entire week before you. Remember that you have to fill this chart every day in the evening. There should be no mistake in this.

You will be more cautious about your eating habits during this week. You will find that you are able to control your desires and inclinations more easily.

Directions—You have to resolve leaving all eating habits that are harmful while filling this chart this week. You have also to take care regarding timings of snacks and meals so that you can have control over them. If your are successful, put in 'A ' fill ' B' if in partial control and 'C' if you have failed to control them.

Second Week

Habit No.	First Day	Second Day	Third Day	Fourth Day	Fifth Day	Sixth Day	Seventh Day
1	A	B	A	A	A	A	A
2	B	A	A	A	A	A	A
3	A	A	A	A	A	A	A
4	A	A	A	A	A	A	A
5	B	B	A	A	B	A	A
6	A	A	B	A	A	A	A
7	A	B	A	A	A	A	A
8	B	A	A	C	A	A	A
9	A	A	A	A	A	A	A
10	B	A	C	A	A	B	A
Total	20	15	15	10	5	5	0

Try to get rid of all bad eating habits and reward yourself when you are able to shake off any of them.

Determine which habit is persisting and you are unable to get rid of it. Now, you have to get rid of it at all costs. For this, evolve some positive rules. For example, if your chart shows that you are still continuing with the habit of munching salted cashew nuts or chocolate or any other snack while viewing television programmes, make a positive rule that you shall not eat anything wRile watching television.

If you still feel like eating more at lunch or dinner time, then you must resolve, "I shall not have second helping of anything during the meals".

Maybe, you still persist in eating with your guests, just to give them company; then make this rule: "I shall apologise to the guests for no~ taking anything and never eat more than what have set for myself."

Reward: Form a habit of rewarding yourself for getting rid of any bad food habit, particularly habits that are difficult to-get rid of. For your success in giving up bad dietary habits, reward yourself with something other than any eatables. You can gift yourself a good book, handkerchieves or some item of clothing like a sari or blouse. After you have changed your habits, try to evaluate the gains of not eating excess food and the worth of things with which you have rewarded yourself. Celebrate your success.

Professor Willi Wriths, Chairman of Max Planck Institute, Dartmund, West Germany, says, "The mothers are responsible for making women fat." He did a survey on 5,000 girls of the age group 14-19. He weighed them, analysed their eating habits and this is what he summarised: "I found that mothers feed their daughters as much as they can. The mothers are extra careful regarding feeding the daughter from childhood. Many of these young girls had a daily intake of 4,000 calories. Such a large intake of calories may be suitable for mine workers, as they have to work really hard. Such excess intake of food not only makes these girls flabby and ill-proportioned, but they also run the risk of spoiling their health. The excess intake of food causes mental dullness. It also gives rise to many health problems."

Reward Plan

Make a list of the things that you like. Do not include any eatables in it. For example, you can include watching television, listening to music, talking to a friend on phone or reading some favourite book or magazine in this list. These things are beneficial.

If you have the habit of munching something now and then, resolve that you will not take anything between breakfast, lunch, afternoon tea or dinner.

Resolve that "I shall not taste anything while cooking them to find if the salt is in proper proportion and the taste is fine". This equally applies to vegetables, meat or fish preparations and all other eatables.

Make a note of the undermentioned rules with your own hand and follow them fully and strictly.

Let the time of eating be as pleasant as possible. Clean the dining table thoroughly. Spread a new table cloth over the table. It would be better if a flower vase adorns the table. In this way, the time of eating will look like a happy event and will not be a dull routine or ritual.

Take care regarding what you eat. Do not be impressed by taste or ingredients. Chew your food properly and do not swallow it hurriedly. If you feel that the food is not tasty, take help of some good cookery book to make it tasty and appetising.

Do not eat and drink simultaneously. First, chew properly whatever you are eating and after swallowing it, then only drink anything.

Try to leave something in the thali o! plate. You will not get any credit marks for cleaning the plate entirely.

Serve yourself a little less in your plate. Lesser than you have been eating so far. If your stomach is full, do not eat anything in excess.

You should not only try to make your food tasty and appetising, but see to it that it looks attractive and inviting.

Leave the evil habit of munching snacks while doing house-hold work. You must give up the habit of eating salted snacks, pastries, fruits, paneer, cashewnuts, groundnuts, chocolates while reading newspaper or talking on phone or while cooking the meals.

You may feel like eating after doing some strenuous work or walking about. This is time of your test. Try to overcome the desire to eat. Postpone eating till proper mealtimes. You can get over the desire to eat by making yourself busy in knitting, combing hair or putting on make-up.

If you are losing weight at a slow pace, do not be disappointed. Remember, your weight increased gradually. You have ample time. Reduction in weight will take some time. Hence, be in a pleasant mood. Do not let this worry you.

Take help from your friends in overcoming your habits. You must choose those friends who tell you positively, "Take care, do not eat anything except at fixed meal times". Avoid such friends, who may say, "why are you eating in between the meals, after deciding not to do so. You are a big fool".

You can do your shopping after. having meals. As your stomach will be full, you will be able to avoid the temptation of eating something in the market. You will not feel like eating anything.

Be happy, as you change your eating habits. Feel contented that you have made these changes to have a healthy body. When you start feeling happy about giving up bad dietary habits, you can be sure that you have given up all habits that contribute to obesity and fatness.

■

24

Yogasanas to Reduce Obesity

Vajrasana (Thunderbolt Posture)

Method—It is named thunderbolt, as it imparts the strength to body as if it is made like a stone or as strong as a thunder bolt. It is the only asana, in yoga, which can be practised after 45 minutes or more from the time of finishing your meals. In between meal times, it can also be done, but never immediately after meals. Kneel down on the floor, letting your big toes, and legs and knees touch the ground. Now rest your buttocks on your knees, your heels bent inwards and thumbs touching each other. Place the palms on the knees, keeping your spine erect but relaxed and flexible. Breathing should be even, deep and slow. Expand your chest, drawing the abdominal muscles inwards.

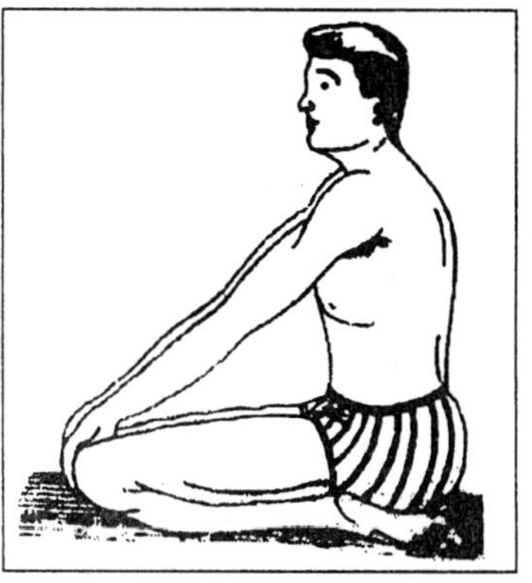

Benefits—This asana will expel gas and remove acidity. How much you have overeating, it will digest the same. It tones up sexual system of both males and females, removes pain and stiffness in spine and knees, lowers raised blood pressure, gives longevity and retards and postpones old age. For meditation, it is an ideal asana, as you can sit in this asana as long as you wish. After completion of this asana, simply massage with your hands or, still better, use salt mixed oil, say of mustard, which can be slightly Luke-warmed.

Dhanurasana (Bow-Shaped Posture)

Method—Lie flat on the ground, your abdominal side touching the ground. Fold your legs from the knees. Now lift your neck and torso, gradually keeping your hands along sides of your back. Try to catch hold of your ankles with your hands. Gradually stretch your hands and feet so that they form a bow-shape, stay in this position as long as you can. Then regain the former position and relax by loosening your limbs.

Benefits—It has all the benefits detailed under Bhujang-asana, as it is simply and extended form of the former. When you are doing Dhanurasana, there is hardly any need for practising Bhujangasana. Its added benefits are in strengthening of hands, elbows, ankles, knees. In short, both the lower and upper extremities become more flexible and strong, abdominal pressure helps in secretion of digestive juice and activities endocrine glands. In both these asanas, no jerk should be exerted on any organ. This suggestion is good for all other asanas too. Pregnant ladies must not perform this asana.

Mandukasana

This asana must have derived its name for the Sanskrit name Manduka which means a frong. Mandukasana does not resemble the frog very much as its name denotes, but the folded legs resemble frog's hind legs and the arms supporting the body look like frog's forelegs. Though this asana looks simple and is also easy to perform, its benefits are plenty.

Method—Kneel down with the knees apart.

Slowly lower the body and sit down between the folded legs in such a way that the buttocks touch the ground. Slowly widen the gap between the knees till they come in a straight line.

Keep the toes close to each other. Lean a little forward and place both the palms near the thighs, fingers turned towards the thighs.

Keep the spine erect, fix your gaze straight and breath normally. Stay so for as long as you can and revert back to original position by releasing the hands first and then drawing in the folded legs together.

Relax and repeat again.

During the initial days of practice, difficulty may be experienced in spreading the legs and it may not come in straight line. The groins may ache if you force it. Gradually, the gap can be decreased without any discomfort.

Benefits—This is a unique exercises for women, teenage girls as well as women of other ages.

All uttering disorders respond well to this exercise. The so-called premenstrual syndrome, like depression, frustration and anxiety can be overcome by practising this asana regularly.

It cures impotence in the males. It strengthens the pelvic muscles and improves circulation in the region.

It helps control bladder and prostate disorders.

Spinal nerves get adequate supply of circulation and they become stronger.

It is a good exercise for obesity too.

Ardhamatsyendrasana

This exercise must be practised by almost every one because this asana and Vakrasana are the asanas that strengthen the spine side ways that too in the vertical position. All other asanas performed lying on the back and abdomen bend the spine forward and backward. Doing Vakrasana first helps doing Ardhamatsyendrasana better and easily.

Method— Sit on the ground and place the left heel under the right thigh.

- Slowly take right leg across the folded left leg and place the foot flat on the ground near the left knee.
- Push the right leg pressing the abdomen by the left hand and place it touching the right foot or hold the right toes.

- Twist the waist towards right and bring your chin in level with your right shoulder.
- Take your right hand behind the back by twisting a little more and touch the right thigh.
- Stay for sometime in this posture and return to original position.
- Repeat the same with the other side.

Benefits—Useful for backache, digestive disorders, liver disorders, diabetes, kidney disorders and for obesity caused due to diabetes and indigestion.

Note—The Asanas explained in the height section can also be practiced alongwith these Asanas.

For more information of Asanas, you should read the book "Pranayama for Better Life" from the same Author and Publisher.

■■■

Other Books on

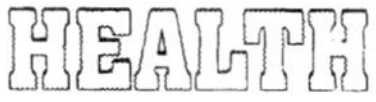

1. A Guide to Your Pregnancy (New)
2. Ayurveda for All (New)
3. A Guide to Migraine, Airthritis, Cervical Spondylosis, and Backache (New)
4. Body and Beauty Care (New)
5. Yoga for All (New)
6. Child Care and Nutrition
7. Naturopathy Modern Way of Life
8. First Aid How to Handle an Accident
9. Acupressure in Daily Life
10. Complete Book of Yoga
11. Look Younger at Any Age
12. HIV/AIDS - Transmission, Prevention and A. Therapies
13. Diabetics and Diet
14. Increase your Height & Loose your Weight
15. Make Fitness A Way of Life
16. Common Problems of Children
17. Handbook of Nutrition & Dietetics
18. A Guide to Massage Therapy
19. A Guide to Family Medicine
20. A Guide to Digestive Disorders
21. Complete Book of Child Care
22. A Guide to Homoeopathy

23. Life Begins at 40
24. Alternative Therapies
25. How to Overcome Stress
26. Yoga Therapy
27. Obesity
28. Self Motivation
29. Yoga for Health and Relaxation
30. Women Disorders and Pregnancy
31. A Guide to Body Pains
32. Sex Education
33. Common Diseases and Cure
34. Pranayama for Better Life
35. Herbal Home Remedies
36. A Guide to Beauty & Skin Care
37. A Guide to Heart Care
38. A Guide to High Blood Pressure
39. Cancer Causes and Prevention
40. Nature Cure for Common Diseases
41. Good Health Through Food and Regimen
42. A Guide to Allergies
43. A Guide to Aging
44. Ayurveda for Health & Beauty

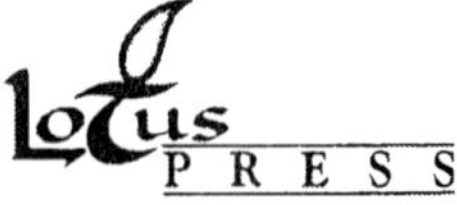